A Nurse and Mother

Also by Evelyn Prentis

A Nurse in Time
A Nurse in Action

A Nurse and Mother

My Life as a Post-War Nurse

EVELYN PRENTIS

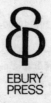

EBURY
PRESS

3 5 7 9 10 8 6 4 2

Published in 2012 by Ebury Press, an imprint of Ebury Publishing
A Random House Group company
First published in Great Britain by
Hutchinson & Co (Publishers) Ltd in 1980

The Random House Group Limited Reg. No. 954009

Addresses for companies within the Random House Group can be
found at www.randomhouse.co.uk

A CIP catalogue record for this book is available from
the British Library

The Random House Group Limited supports The Forest Stewardship
Council (FSC®), the leading international forest certification organisa-
tion. Our books carrying the FSC label are printed on FSC® certified
paper. FSC is the only forest certification scheme endorsed by the leading
environmental organisations, including Greenpeace. Our paper procure-
ment policy can be found at www.randomhouse.co.uk/environment

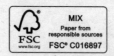

Printed and bound by CPI Group (UK) Ltd, Croydon, CR0 4YY

ISBN 9780091941383

To buy books by your favourite authors and register for offers visit
www.randomhouse.co.uk

For my sons-in-law
From me

Part One

Part One

Chapter One

THE WAR WAS over. It had taken two curtain calls before it finally came to an end, the second more final and more dramatic than the first.

When we heard the news about the bomb on Hiroshima the event was too distant to have us trembling with fear as some of us had done while our own bombs were falling around us. The shock waves that resulted from it took a long time to travel from Japan, and when they eventually reached us I was one of the many who secretly wondered whether enough good had come out of the evil to justify it. It was a question we were to ponder over and argue about for a long time, without getting any nearer an answer that would satisfy all our doubts. But at least the bomb brought the war to an uneasy end, which even I had to admit was a blessing, however much I disliked the way the blessing was disguised.

The first Victory Day was a splendid affair; an occasion for rejoicing unmarred by lingering doubts, vain soul-searchings or sleep-disturbing guilt complexes. A time for the lifting of the blackout and the raising of hopes that tomorrow – and all the tomorrows thereafter – would be perfect. They weren't but the thought that they might be kept the people dancing in the streets and falling into fountains far into the night, determined in the shortest possible time to make up for the dreariness of the past six years. Children were put into fancy dresses and funny paper hats, flags were found and frantically waved and jealously hoarded jellies were produced from the backs of dark cupboards to be cunningly transformed into wobbly rabbits or castles on the point of collapse, adding blobs of watery colour to the Union-Jack-draped trestle tables and making the children's eyes grow round with the wonder of it all. It was the first chance most of them had had for such unbridled gluttony and would perhaps be the last for a long time to come. Though the war was as good as over rationing was still with us; coupons were almost as important as money, and there were quarrelsome queues for potatoes.

I might have made a paper hat myself or even a wobbly rabbit but for the fact that my infant daughter was still at an age where anything weightier than a woolly bonnet would have sat uneasily on her silky head, and the thought of the harm a spoonful of jelly might do to her tender tummy was enough to make me tremble. It may have done no harm at all, but I had been a nurse for too long to think of exposing her to such a terrible risk. I kept strictly to the rules I had been taught to keep in hospital and fed my child, and later my children, with the right and proper things, which didn't include extras like jelly while they were still at the dried milk stage. I also turned a deaf ear to their pleading when they tried to tell me they were hungry less than five minutes before their next feed was due. I knew that such childish rebellion had to be put down from the start if they were ever to become balanced and responsible adults. Both my children were going on for twenty before I discovered Dr Spock and learned how sadly I had mismanaged the whole thing. By denying them the luxury of feeds on demand, total exemption from potty training and uninhibited self-expression I had done untold damage to their emotional development. But it was too late then. What was done was done.

I brooded over it while I was drinking a cup of tea one morning, and then put the Spock book back on the shelf and comforted myself with the thought that millions of mothers past and present had brought up their families without guidance from the good doctor and seemed to have made a reasonably good job of it. But I still watched anxiously for signs of emotional damage. I kept remembering the hours I had made them sit on potties and the scoldings I gave them if the result of the sitting hadn't justified the bright red rings they wore almost permanently around their dimpled little bottoms.

As well as not making a paper hat or a wobbly rabbit I didn't dance in the street or fall into a fountain throughout the entire Victory celebrations, though I lost at least one of my inhibitions before the revelling was over. When my neighbours came knocking on my door and invited me to a party they were having I told them that I was teetotal and didn't go to parties. I didn't bother to explain that the main reason I didn't go to parties was because I never got asked. Or at least I never got asked a second time. Being strictly teetotal had always been something of a drawback to me on festive occasions, or on any other occasion that called for a little loosening of the inhibitions. I didn't loosen easily, which made me less than an asset at any informal gathering that depended on more than a cup of tea for its success.

But the neighbours who knocked at my door refused to take no for an answer to their invitation and at last, much against my better judgement, I bundled my sleeping angel into several shawls, put her in her pram and went next door, already dreading the debauchery I knew I would be faced with when I got there. We parked the pram in the pram-packed kitchen and went into the front room where the party was in full swing. I was greatly relieved when somebody offered me a glass of orange juice. It was only after the glass had been refilled twice that it began to dawn on me that the orange juice I was drinking had a subtly different flavour from the juice that was handed out to us every week at the Welfare Clinic. The headache I woke up with the next morning told me beyond all doubt that my teetotal days were over; it also made me vow never to drink more than two glasses of anything that looked like orange juice but tasted subtly different. I didn't always keep the vow but I never broke it enough to get more than a headache the following morning, and after years of being strictly teetotal I was forced to admit that the party I went to on Victory night was the best I had ever been to.

Soon after the bomb was dropped on Hiroshima the servicemen began pouring off the trains clutching their final travel warrants in their hands and looking very dapper in their chalk-striped demob suits. The home-coming wasn't always the ecstatic reunion they had dreamed about while they were away. Returning husbands who had grown accustomed over the years to the comradeship of danger often found themselves missing the comradeship, some even missed the danger. Those who had dreamed of civvy street from a long way off were amazed how drab civvy street could look when viewed from one of its terraced houses. And however fearful the encounters with the enemy or the

Regimental Sergeant Major had been, the encounters with the clerks behind the desk at the labour exchange were never the happy little get-togethers that had been promised the war-weary men. There were pinpricks which if less painful than bullet wounds could still cause a lot of discomfort.

Neither were the wives always as jubilant as they had expected to be once they had their man about the house again. Those who had become proficient at unblocking a sink in minutes were apt to grow tetchy with husbands who spent hours on their hands and knees searching for a stopcock, especially when the result of the search was a pool of water on the newly scrubbed kitchen floor and a sink as blocked as it had been before the search began. Many a wife had gone right through the war without a stopcock. Some didn't know that such a thing existed. A knitting needle long enough to poke down the plug hole and some hot water with a lump of common soda dissolved in it were all they ever needed to dislodge whatever was lodged in the pipes. But it was a waste of time trying to tell a demobbed husband this. He had just come out of the army, the navy or the air force. He knew all the scientific ways of dealing with blocked-up sinks. He threw scorn on the bucket of soda water and spurned the offer of a knitting needle, however unsuccessful his scientific methods turned out to be.

Nor were the children immune from it all. Those who had been warned what life with father would be like unless they mended their ways and crept round the house like mice when he came home hadn't looked forward to having him home. The ogre with the belt they had so often been threatened with loomed menacingly in the background, making it hard for father to change his image however loving he set out to be. Not every father had the patience to go on being patient in the teeth of his children's hostility. Some gave up trying and became the ogre with the belt instead.

Even the babies didn't find the war-to-peace transition easy. Those who had heard no other sound in the night but the soft murmur of their mother's voice took instant fright when a strange harsh voice came out of the darkness. They also took umbrage. Though they couldn't possibly have understood a word of what was being said in the dark, their instinct told them that none of it was being said to them. By the same sixth sense they were able to deduce that none of what was currently being done in the dark was being done for their benefit. Suddenly having to take a back seat in the house where for so long they had been the central character caused them uncontrollable grief. They gave vent to their grief with fits of screaming which left the neighbours in no doubt that they were being murdered. The screams caused as many rifts between frustrated husband and anxious mother as they did between resentful father and furiously jealous baby; they had a tendency to break out at the most inconvenient moment.

It was usually while I was feeding the pig-bin with my household scraps that I heard of the post-war problems that were besetting my neighbours. We lived in a tiny terraced house not far from the house where we had first lodged when we got married. Nance, our landlady, had startled me one day by telling me that she was going to be divorced. Until then I had only read about divorce in the newspapers. Nobody I knew had ever done anything as daring. If any of my married acquaintances found themselves growing a little disillusioned with their partner they kept quiet about it and went on lying on the lumpy bed they had made for themselves, getting what comfort they could from it, or they continued living with the lumps for the sake of the children. Nance had no children, which was perhaps one of the reasons for her refusal to put up with the lumps any longer.

It was Nance who had helped me to find the small house and had let us have a few bits of furniture and a mat or two at a price which she assured us were well below their market value. She had also kindly offered to help me with the distempering. She said that reaching up wasn't good for somebody in my condition: it could get the cord round the baby's neck quicker than anything. Since the baby was due any minute, it was a matter of supreme importance that nothing dire should befall it. Nance distempered the whole house in a shocking shade of pink, then went over it all again with a piece of lace curtain which she dipped into a bucket of distemper of a darker shade of pink and dabbed it across the walls. She said it was called stippling and assured me it was the latest thing in interior decorating. It was a lot cheaper than wall-paper, she said. When I suggested timidly that maybe the walls should have been stripped of the old paper before the new distemper was applied she reminded me tartly that she was doing the job, and if I thought I could do it any better she would be quite happy to stand aside and watch while I put the baby's future in jeopardy by getting the cord entangled. I mixed another bucket of distemper and tried not to think of my mother's frenzied attacks on the walls in the spring and autumn.

When my husband came home to the little terraced house for his first long leave he didn't take kindly to the shocking pink background, or to the lace-curtain dabbed cabbages that ran amok across every wall. After he had gone twice through his repertoire of bad language suitable to be used in front of a woman he tore into the town and bought packets of distemper of a less vivid colour and a proper distemper brush. He worked non-stop throughout his leave and, at the end of it, though the blotches could still be faintly discerned, they were at least a little easier to live with. He went back to camp a tired man, ready for the comparative leisure of square bashing, picket duties and brisk marches round the perimeter. He had only just gone when the bump that I had been carrying round under my smock for nine long months went slowly and painfully down and our first daughter was born.

The pig-bin was shared by all the other houses in the terrace. Every day a farmer drove up, hoisted the bin on to his cart, replaced it with another and went off with our contributions to the obesity of his pigs. The pig-bin played an important part in the war-effort; it was also a popular meeting place for airing views, commiserating happily with the woes of a mutual friend or rejoicing sadly over the downfall of a common enemy.

Until the Victory-night party when I had been accepted by my neighbours and proved to them that I wasn't as stand-offish as they had always thought I was, the founder members of the discussion group at the pig-bin had stood in tight lipped silence waiting for me to go away before they continued with what they were saying before I arrived on the scene. From the way their voices tailed off when I got within earshot I could only conclude that I was the chosen topic for the day.

The suspicion was confirmed after I became a group member. I quickly learned that when one was there we ran down one who wasn't and when the other was there we picked on the absent one. The circle was wide but seldom vicious.

Many of the problems that were discussed over the potato peelings seemed trivial and easily solved to those who didn't have to solve them. Those who did were sometimes thrown into despair by them. When Edna who lived at the top of the terrace told us about her son who had started cheeking his father, Selina from down the other end saw nothing in the situation to get alarmed about. 'All he needs is a clip round the ear'ole,' she said, throwing a shovel full of red hot cinders into the pig-bin. We were not allowed to throw cinders in the bin but Selina lived by her own rules.

'It's easy for you to talk,' said Edna in a defeated way. 'You don't have to put up with it. Besides he's fifteen and bigger than his dad. He wouldn't stand still long enough to be clipped round the ear'ole.' Selina slammed the lid down on the smoking bin and stormed off leaving a strong smell of burning cabbage stalks behind her.

Neither size nor age had ever been things to be reckoned with in her house. That she was their mother raised her in stature far above her sons, whatever age and however tall they were. She had brought up six boys, clipping them round the ear'ole whenever she thought they would benefit from it. Each of them was a credit to her.

When Edna's son came to an inevitable bad end, Selina said she had always said he would, then she went off to do what she could to comfort poor Edna.

Dilys was the first in the terrace to show signs of cracking up under the strain of the armistice. This delighted Edna. She and Dilys were sworn enemies. They had quarrelled over something so long ago that neither of them could remember what it was they had quarrelled about but they hadn't spoken to each other since. They turned their heads and looked pointedly in opposite directions whenever they came within snubbing distance.

Dilys was a well-built girl. She had a pair of sturdy knees that rubbed together when she walked. Her legs had a purple mottling from being huddled too close to the fire in winter and despite her youth they were already knotted with varicose veins caused by a serious weight problem. While the war was on she had spent her days sorting out ration-book problems in the local food office and her nights dreaming of her soldier husband who should have been snoring beside her instead of somewhere in the middle of Salisbury Plain cooking terrible meals for his battalion. Now that the war was over and he had been demobbed,

Dilys still worked in the food office by day but her nights hadn't quite come up to her expectations, or rather we gathered they had surpassed her wildest dreams.

At first we were unaware of the havoc that peace had brought to Dilys's love life. For a day or two after the reunion she had kept us enthralled with a blow by blow account of the breathtaking variations on a similar theme that her lusty young husband had thought up for their mutual delight the night before. Some of the gymnastic feats she described to us could only have been performed at the risk of damaging something and, with a figure like Dilys's, none of them could have been easy. But, as Edna said spitefully after we had been left marvelling: 'Her husband being an army cook all them years he's probably used to humping bloody great sacks of potatoes about.'

Edna had a daughter as well as a no-good son. The daughter was as thin as a rake and had been loosely engaged to a Scottish Highlander since the night right at the beginning of the war when he put his hand on her knee in the pictures. She was still waiting for the invitation to go to Scotland to meet his family. We of the discussion group had decided long ago that the closest family he was likely to have would be his own sons and daughters, and he wouldn't be too eager to invite Edna's daughter to meet them, especially if their mother happened to be around when the meeting was planned. It took Edna a long time to face up to the fact that her daughter's Highlander was never going to marry her. When he stopped sending a card at Christmas we felt very sorry for Edna: we realized she'd lost a lot of face. We felt sorry for the deserted daughter as well.

Selina expressed our sympathy in a few well-chosen words. 'I should forget about him if I were you,' she said cheerfully. 'It's as I've always said, good riddance to bad rubbish, and there's as good a fish in the sea as ever came out of it.' She paused for a moment and looked thoughtful. 'I don't suppose she ever got the chance to look up his kilt either, which is a pity.'

Edna's daughter eventually married someone else, but he was in a wheelchair at thirty and dead by forty. After that she came home to live with her mother and didn't get married again. Neither did she ever put on any weight.

It was only a week or so after Dilys's husband was demobbed that she startled us with her outburst. We were all in Selina's house when it happened. She had asked us in for a cup of tea. 'Come informal,' she'd said, as if we were in the habit of climbing into a ballgown to partake of a cup of tea.

We were halfway through our second chocolate finger – Selina had a friend who worked in the Maypole and could occasionally get hold of a few extras without having to surrender coupons for them – when somebody asked Dilys if she was feeling all right. She had been looking a bit pale lately and not her usual happy self. To everybody's horror Dilys put her cup and plate down on the floor and burst into tears. We looked away. None of us had seen Dilys in tears before, and we were not prepared for the sight.

'It's him,' she gulped after she had blown her nose on the handkerchief that somebody hastily drew from a knitting bag. We pricked up our ears. We could only assume that she was referring to her husband and any disclosures she made about him were bound to be interesting.

'What about him?' asked Selina searching round for another handkerchief.

'He never gives over,' sniffed Dilys sadly. 'It's last thing at night, first thing in the morning. I don't mind telling you I've just about had enough of it.' She yawned widely leaving us to hazard a guess at what she'd just about had enough of. There were no prizes offered for guessing correctly.

Selina got up from her chair and went across to the sofa. 'There now, don't fret, Dill,' she said kindly, patting Dilys's hand. 'After all, considering all he went without while he was away he probably thinks he's got a right to do a bit of catching up.' Selina was always telling us how she'd given that sort of thing up after she'd started the change. She'd had to put her foot down very firmly in bed she told us.

Some of us had doubts about the duration of Dilys's husband's celibacy but we nibbled our fingers and said nothing.

'Well, all right I'll grant you that,' conceded Dilys yawning again, even more cavernously. 'But he surely didn't have to catch up with it all in one week, did he?'

There were nods of sympathetic agreement from some of her listeners, mostly from those who had taken comfort from snuggling down with a good book after the sleeping partners had forsaken the marriage bed to answer the call of duty. When the time came for the book to be laid aside in favour of other pursuits it hadn't always been easy to switch from a little light reading to a lot of heavy breathing.

Dilys lost more sleep and even a little weight adjusting to the switch. She only went back to being her old fat happy self when she told us she was expecting and her mother had said it might be twins seeing as there were twins on her father's side. It was twins. They were fat and happy just like Dilys. They kept their parents far too busy in the night making feeds and changing nappies to leave much time for anything else. But they were worth all the sacrifices he was having to make for them, said Dilys's husband proudly, as he pushed the pram his mother had given them in honour of the twins being her first grandchildren.

Even Edna had to admit the babies were lovely. She started knitting little pink and blue things and soon she and Dilys were the best of friends, their hatchets buried, their differences forgotten.

I had my own post-war problems but none of them as noteworthy as Edna's or Dilys's. I went on reading in bed after my airman husband came home but chose books from the library that could be put down without losing the thread. I continued to unblock the sink with a knitting needle and a handful of soda thrown into a bucket of water, but I was happy to get help with lighting the fires. I wasn't good at lighting fires. However carefully I arranged paper and sticks, and however many matches I applied to the arrangement the results were invariably the same – a crackling great flame shooting straight up the chimney, then nothing and the whole process to be gone through again. Once, disheartened by successive pyrogenic failures, I threw a can of paraffin on the smouldering sticks, but the flames shot out instead of up and I amazed my friends for a long time with a jagged fringe and no eyebrows.

There were other things I wasn't terribly efficient at. Being a nurse had not given me a light hand with pastry or a sure touch with a sewing needle. I could have whipped round a ward with a trolley full of bedpans in less time than it took me to attach a button to a shirt. Not one of the sponge cakes I made after I got married weighed an ounce less than the linseed poultices I slapped on the patients while I was doing my training. I got into a greater muddle with the household accounts than I did with the complicated sums that used to have to be done to work out the required dosage of a dangerous drug. Being a nurse had not prepared me for the tragedies and disasters of being a housewife. I wept bitter tears over the apple pie that slipped through my scorched fingers and landed upside down in a squashy heap on the hearth. I watched with heavy heart as my cakes sank slowly in the middle, and I shrieked with hysteria when a mouse pattered across the kitchen floor. Though I had seen a million cockroaches congregated together in a hospital kitchen they were as nothing to the one solitary mouse that careered across my own kitchen floor.

Nurses learn many things while they are training to be nurses but little of what they learn is of much practical help when an apple pie falls to the ground only seconds before it is due to be dished up, or when a well-sprung mouse trap needs to be baited with cheese. Knowing how to give an enema is no substitute for not knowing how to turn a sheet sides to middle. The mysteries of housework gave me as many headaches as had the mysteries of anatomy and physiology when I was grappling with them. As with the anatomy and physiology, many of the finer points of housework were to remain a mystery to me for ever.

Chapter Two

HOWEVER GRIEVOUS WAS the tragedy of the apple pie, there was an even greater tragedy to follow. If the catastrophe of the sunken cakes had been no act of God, the floods that came to ruin many of our fixtures and fittings most certainly were. They followed a bleak and bitter winter that sent the fuel bills soaring almost into double figures and made bed the warmest place to be in, though even bed wasn't always proof against the icy blast which didn't take long to find its way through a utility blanket.

There were two children to share the floods with us. The second, fitting nicely into her sister's shrunken woollies, gave me the chance to boast about 'my daughters' with the utmost satisfaction.

The flood waters rose rapidly. One minute they were a silver shimmer in the distance between two rivers swollen with melting snow and lashing rain, the next they were across the road and we were awash. Soon there were waves lapping the table legs and creeping along the carpet. A chair leg floated, a cupboard door fell off, stuffing oozed wetly from beneath the sofa and a mat fell to pieces before our eyes, proving how right Nance had been to undercut the junk shops with her few mats and bits and pieces of furniture.

My husband paddled home from work and splashed into the living room, where I stood on a table with a wriggling child under each arm. He joined me on the table and we clung together waiting for rescue to come.

The man who volunteered to rescue me was of less than average height and well below bantam weight. He looked as if another inch or two of flood water would have totally submerged him. He waded in, his thigh-high boots making terrible squelching noises as he walked, did a quick calculation of my body weight, greatly enlarged with two babies and too many apple pies, then braced himself. 'You'll have to straddle me back,' he said, sounding not too keen on the idea. Any hopes I might have had of being swept up in a pair of manly arms, in the way that the women in *Gone with the Wind* were always being swept up, went with the wind. I straddled the poor little man's back and after one or two false starts made a less than dignified exit from my waterlogged home.

Going back there again after the waters went down was a sorry business. The lower floors were encrusted with mud, and a dado of inky slime marked where the high water line had been. Streaks of rising damp rose almost to the ceiling and the paper on the walls, which Nance and I should have torn off, now hung in soggy ribbons. Again I wept, but for more than a shattered pie crust. I wept for what I then foolishly thought was the worst blow that life could deal us.

'Put it down to experience,' said my husband philosophically as we were shovelling up the mud. I tried but it still hurt. It went on hurting for a long time. The sofa was never the same again.

After the floods came chicken pox, measles and whooping cough, all in quick succession and all in duplicate. The chicken pox and measles we could have lived without but the whooping cough was very much worse, especially in duplicate. At least with the earlier scourges there had been a short breathing space between one child throwing off her final itchy spot or scab and the other catching it, but with the whooping cough there was no such respite. Hardly were we back in bed after swinging the youngest by her heels to save her from choking than there came a terrible whoop from her sister's cot and the whole terrifying cycle began again.

We sent for the doctor, but he told us that it would have to run its course and suggested that we bought a bottle of cough mixture from the chemist. He didn't call again. He might have been a little more attentive if we hadn't fallen a week or two behind with our contributions to a family medical scheme. We should have paid a shilling a week with unfailing regularity but a shilling was a lot to lay out unless you could be reasonably certain that somebody was going to be ill enough to benefit from it. We hadn't reckoned on chicken pox, measles and whooping cough all in quick succession and all in duplicate. If we had we would most certainly have willingly handed over our shilling, instead of pretending we were out when the collector called.

Because the neighbours had discovered that I was a nurse before I became a mother, they expected me to have some miracle cure for the coughs that racked our children and wrecked our nights. I had no such cure. Being a nurse didn't help at all; it only made things worse. I knew from experience that children could die of the simplest things, even of something as simple as whooping cough. I had watched them die while their mothers stood at their cot sides praying for them to live. Prayer wasn't always enough to clear a path through congested lungs and choked-up throats. I remembered one terrible night when I was doing my training. The ambulance had brought in a child with whooping cough. He was a beautiful boy. His mother was older than most mothers of children of his age. She had waited a long time for him, and when he arrived he was the answer to all her hopes and dreams. She refused to believe that the same God who had given her

her son was about to rob her of him. Her prayers for his life were not answered. Immunization and antibiotics came too late for her child; until such things became available to everybody we dosed our children with useless cough mixtures and went on praying that they would reach the climax of a whoop and start breathing properly again before it was too late.

Selina knocked on the door one morning to enquire how the children were. I had invited her in, and she kindly offered to pass on to me some remedies for whooping cough which she assured me were never known to fail. They only failed that day because we didn't have any of the things that the remedies required to make them a success.

'We need a bit of hot tar,' she said, as she held one child's head over a wash bowl while I pounded the other on the back. 'A bit of hot tar would get right down into their lungs and do the trick in no time.'

'Where would we find hot tar?' I asked, not because I had any faith in it as a remedy but simply because I had got to the point where I would have welcomed a whole cauldron of tar in my sitting room if it would only have stopped the children coughing.

'It's a pity there isn't a bit of road works going on somewhere in the vicinity,' said Selina. I could think of no road works going on in the vicinity and neither could she.

'What about the gas works?' I said. 'There would be some hot tar there, perhaps.' I didn't know whether there would be hot tar at the gas works or not but I stopped wondering about it when I remembered that the nearest gasometer was ten miles away.

Selina went off to empty the wash bowl ready for the next bout of coughing to fill it again. She came back with another card up her sleeve.

'Taking them up in an aeroplane would be the next best thing,' she said. I looked at her over the youngest's navy blue face. The youngest must have beaten all records for the length of time she held her breath during a spasm of coughing. The idea of taking them up in an aeroplane was as far fetched as suddenly coming across a cauldron of hot tar behind the kitchen door. Despite the glories of the Battle of Britain, and all the things that Mr Churchill had said about the many owing so much to the few, the many were still not too blasé about aeroplanes. A single one flying over the rooftops could have us staring at the sky with interest. There wasn't the remotest chance of getting our poor little whoopers up in an aeroplane. I waited for Selina's next infallible cure for whooping cough. I didn't have to wait long.

'Goose-grease,' she exclaimed suddenly. 'My poor old mother used to swear by goose-grease when we were kids. She always kept a basinful of it in the larder and when any of us had a chesty cough she used to spread some on a bit of old flannel, slap it on and leave it to soak it in. It worked like a charm.'

Under my close interrogation Selina admitted that her poor old mother hadn't sworn by goose-grease for a long time. Succulent roast goose wasn't a regular feature of anybody's diet and without the goose there could be no basinful of grease in the larder ready to be slapped on at the first croak or wheeze.

'Oh well, not to worry,' she said, grinning. 'It's perhaps just as well there isn't any. It used to smell terrible after it had been soaking in for a day or two. Nobody would sit next to us at school when we had a cough.'

She went off home and I resigned myself to more sleepless nights and more terrifying moments waiting for the youngest to draw breath again.

Like the flood waters the coughs gradually went away, leaving none of us unscathed by the experience. The children were pale and sickly and we were weary after so many broken nights.

'Do you think we should take them to visit your parents for a few days?' my husband said, with an annual holiday due. I tossed and turned throughout the night in an agony of doubt as to whether or not the effort of taking two young children on the many-trained journey from the outskirts of London to the depths of Lincolnshire would be worth whatever benefit they might get from it. In the morning I looked at their small pale faces, remembered the abundance of fresh air that abounded where my parents lived and started making plans for the holiday.

The very small smallholding where I had spent most of my childhood had changed little over the years. When the war came it swept like a flurrying wind over cottage, barn and pigsty, leaving no trace that it had ever been there except for the patches of milk-white arabis, or snow-in-the-mountains as the country folk call it, which the soldiers had planted and left as a perennial memorial to their temporary occupation of my father's field. The little brook ran as it had always run, beside the house, past the nettle-bedded privy and on through the gorse bushes in the paddock. Trains rumbled by puffing white smoke and whistling an amiable greeting to the level-crossing keeper. The Co-op man called on Thursday but in a motorized vehicle now and not the horse-drawn covered wagon that had made Thursday so special when I was a child and left us with a warm and pungent top dressing to put on the rhubarb. The horse had been a creature of habit. It never failed to deliver the top dressing while it waited patiently for the Co-op man to deliver the groceries.

My mother washed on Monday, did the bedrooms on Tuesday, relentlessly scrubbed and polished on Wednesday and again on Thursday, baked on Friday, prepared the Sunday dinner on Saturday and went to church twice every Sunday. If it were ever possible for time to stand still, then it almost certainly stood still in the little house down the lane and up the cart track where we were planning on taking the children to convalesce after the winter of floods, chicken pox, measles and whooping cough.

The plans had to be made with meticulous attention to detail. Though we had done the journey with both children in their infancy, taking two at the walking stage required considerable forethought. We bought shoes and socks with the rent money, paid the rent with the coal money and didn't answer the door when the coalman came knocking. With fares to pay and sundries to buy there was nothing left for him in the tin marked 'coalman' which we kept on the shelf beside the tin marked 'milkman'. In the hope of softening the blow a little we dropped a note through his letter box apologizing for being out when he called and promising payment in full the next time we saw him. We were pleasantly surprised when he didn't rush round at once to re-claim what was left of the last lot he delivered. We had never owed the coalman money before; we didn't know what steps he would take.

The holiday was lovely. There was as much fresh air as anybody could have wished for. The children sniffed it in noisily realizing that it had a different smell from the air they were used to sniffing in. My mother smiled indulgently while they did things that I would have been smacked for doing when I was their age and my father called them his little birdies and doted on them. Neither of them fell down the well in the garden, though they lived dangerously teetering on the edge looking for the toad that their grandfather told them lived down there. He had told me the same story when I was a child, but I never saw the toad. He said that every well needed a toad to purify the water. It had always seemed to me to be an odd way of purifying water but certainly not as complicated as the sewage system I had to learn about after I became a nurse.

When we walked down the lane to fetch the milk from a neighbouring farm the children squealed with delight as the farmer squirted them with fresh warm milk straight from the cow and roared with anger when his little boy mocked them and called them Cockneys. Neither of them knew what a Cockney was, but it sounded nasty enough to bring out the fighting spirit in them. The war was brought to an end by the kind farmer's wife who took the two little Cockneys with her while she collected the eggs and gave them a brown one each for their tea.

They walked back up the cart track swinging the milk can round and round and from side to side, almost churning the contents to butter before it was delivered safely to the cool dark larder. Swinging the milk can round was one of the things I was never allowed to do when I was a child, but my mother said it was different for them – they got milk from a bottle and not from a cow. Swinging the can round also took their minds off their aching feet. Like me they were more used to riding on buses than walking down long lanes and up rutted cart tracks.

It was after they were in bed that night and while we were eating our bread and cheese and drinking our thick, sweet cocoa that my mother broke a habit of a lifetime. She mentioned sex. Except for the heavily veiled warnings she had given me the day before I left home to be a nurse about what could happen to me if I wasn't a good girl she had given no indication at all that she knew such a thing as sex existed. So what had made that night different from all others I never knew unless it was the memory of the farmer squirting the children with the fresh warm milk.

'Cows don't need bulls these days,' she said, pouring more sugar into my father's cocoa. 'They get injections instead.' And that was it. We learned nothing more from her about the miracle of AID that was just beginning to hit the headlines in the *Farmer's Weekly*. My father speared the last bit of red cheddar on to his knife and avoided my eye. He had no intention of making any contribution to the loose talk that was threatening to sully the supper table.

At the end of the holidays we went home with two rosy-cheeked children, four plump ducks and a rusty old bicycle.

The ducks were my father's idea. He had the deepest contempt for men who earned their living without getting their hands dirty. 'Pen pusher,' he growled scornfully when my office-based husband showed us the blisters he had won for weather proofing the porch over the gnarled old kitchen door, painting everything paintable inside and outside the house and sawing up enough tree trunks to keep my parents' home fires burning until the next time we visited them. When we told him about the fair-sized garden that went with the house we lived in his eyes lit up. He saw it at once as a means of redeeming at least a few of his son-in-law's decadent city ways, or at least of getting his hands soiled occasionally.

'You should start a smallholding,' he said, blowing smoke rings to delight the children and gently stroking the flaxen head of the youngest.

We tried to tell him that starting a smallholding with a plot of ground no bigger than his cabbage patch, in the middle of a fairly well built-up area, might not be easy, but he was not to be discouraged by such trifling details.

'You'd have to start small,' he said, separating the children who had started a major dispute over whose turn it was to blow out the next match.

The ducks we took home with us were to be the nucleus of the smallholding my father had dreamed up for us, but they didn't live long enough to make his dreams come true.

The bicycle was my mother's contribution towards our future well being. From the time I left home to be a nurse it had hung from a hook in the barn gathering red rust. Both the tyres were flat and generations of mice had made their home in the saddlebag.

My husband put up a lot of resistance against being lumbered with the bicycle but my mother was adamant. She pointed out that it would be useful for me to ride to church on. I didn't tell her that I only went to church at Christmas and Easter, on special occasions like weddings and christenings, and to the funeral of somebody I had liked well enough to mourn. I only ever told my mother the things I thought she would want to hear, and she certainly wouldn't have wanted to hear about my lapse from grace. She had brought me up to bike to church twice every Sunday and to choir practice during the week. That the seeds she had so carefully sown had failed to bear fruit was something which I thought best to conceal from her.

After a brave attempt at arguing with her, my

husband sullenly tied labels on the bicycle and arranged for it to be stowed away in the guard's van with the crate of ducks. It had taken him a long time to learn that when my mother was adamant she remained adamant in the teeth of the most determined opposition. It was a hard lesson for him to learn. He also had his adamant moments. On the occasions that his and hers clashed there were enough sparks to set light to the barn.

The journey home was made memorable by a small incident that took place while we were travelling in a taxi from one side of London to the other. (We had pooled what was left of our holiday money and, with a copper or two that the children reluctantly handed over, managed to scrape enough together to cover the fare. We tried not to think of the coalman going bankrupt while he waited another week for his money.) The cab driver was a family man himself, he told us, looking fondly at the children, and had often thought of keeping a bit of poultry in his own back yard in Bow, he said, looking with envy at the ducks. He piled the children, us and the hand luggage into the cab, then stood and scratched his ear while he thought what to do with the bike and the ducks.

'They'd better be shoved on top,' he bawled at us through the cab window. Shoving them on top took several minutes. It should perhaps have taken longer. At the first confrontation with another vehicle the taxi pulled up sharply, there was a slithering noise from above and the passengers on the top deck made a rapid descent to the road below.

The crate that my father had knocked up in a hurry hadn't been designed to take such a sudden shock. It burst open at all seams and one by one the ducks stepped out, quacked with joy at their sudden freedom and waddled across the road looking for a muddy pond or some other familiar landmark. Horns honked, brakes squealed and traffic came to a standstill. Every passing pedestrian joined in the chase and even the bus drivers climbed down from their high perches and flapped wildly.

When the corralling was finally over the cab driver made us sit holding the crate on our laps while he proceeded at a very slow pace to the underground station.

We ate the ducks one by one, using the next four Sundays as excuses for the orgies and much later we went out and bought four young pullets, but though they laid plenty of free-range eggs for us they never became a smallholding.

Chapter Three

FOR THE NEXT few years our lives lacked any great excitement. My father-in-law came to live with us, but not, alas, for long. He and I were comfortable together in the warm friendship that had sprung up between us on my wedding day when he was invited to accompany the groom and me on our honeymoon. He had travelled from the far north to the deep south to witness his only son being married, and the thought of him turning round and making the weary journey back home again, with the bombs falling and the blackout making travelling difficult, saddened the day for all us. It took time to persuade him to make up a threesome on a honeymoon, but he had at last given in and accepted the invitation though not without some bewilderment and a few canny Tyneside observations.

Since the honeymoon was spent at my mother's, where the sleeping arrangements were already cramped with evacuees, it never properly became a honeymoon. My mother had insisted on her new son-in-law sharing the guest room with his father while I was tucked in with the evacuees. But at least my father-in-law enjoyed it. He saw more of his son in one week than he had seen since the war began, or would see again until he came to live out his last few months with us.

We were desolate when he died. Even the children mourned for him, missing his gentle finger on their cheek and the sound of his voice as he gave us 'The Blaydon Races' and other Northumbrian ditties sung *fortissimo*.

Discovering that I was a nurse had not only given the neighbours the idea that I could work miracles with whooping cough, it had fostered in them the belief that I was an authority on all things medical and a fount of wisdom when advice was sought. It took them a while to reconcile themselves to the fact that I was neither. They described symptoms that I had no explanation for and expected me to come up with an immediate diagnosis of the tortures that had kept them awake all night. They also hurled stones at my bedroom window in the middle of the night if their babies had teething problems, or if something more serious had thrown them into sad chaos.

The first time something like this happened I edged my way from under the blankets with extreme caution, taking care not to disturb my sleeping husband. He needed a full eight hours of oblivion before he was in any shape to face another day. Neighbours throwing stones at the bedroom window did not immediately arouse him to a compassionate understanding of their needs.

'Who is it?' I called out, throwing open the window and letting in a cold front followed by a sudden blast of squally rain. It was a very nasty night.

'It's me,' answered a voice from below.

Whoever it was I didn't recognize the voice, neither did I recognize the woman who was standing on my doorstep. I went downstairs and unbolted the door.

'Are you the nurse that lives here?' asked the woman straining to get a better look at me through the darkness.

I confessed to being a nurse and living there, then I asked her what I could do for her. I hoped it wasn't much. I also needed sleep to knit the ravelled sleeve of care.

'It's Grandma,' said the woman. 'We think she's gone. We wondered whether you'd mind coming and having a look at her for us. If it's not too much to ask, that is.'

For a moment it was much too much to ask. There was something in the invitation to go and have a look at a grandma who might be gone that brought to mind all I had ever read of a gin-soaked Mrs Gamp reeling out in the night to deal incompetently with an emergency case. Though I hadn't touched a drop since Victory night, having my hair in curlers and my feet in an old pair of carpet slippers did nothing to soften the image. But almost at once the professional instinct that lies deeply rooted in the heart of all nurses, whether born or otherwise, took over. I went back upstairs and gave my husband a few useful tips on how to cope for an hour or two without me, then removed the slippers and curlers, put on a raincoat and a pair of wellington boots and went with the woman.

The extremely old lady who was lying in a bed upstairs had indeed gone. A considerable time must have elapsed from the moment that help should have been fetched to the moment when I arrived on the scene. I worked hard for a long time with only the light from a guttering candle to work by. Grandma's room was basic, lacking the refinement of an electric light bulb. It also lacked certain other things that would have made my task easier. The water in the bowl on the marble wash-hand stand was almost as cold as the old lady had become.

When all was finished I went downstairs. The little group standing round the empty grate in the living room shuffled uncomfortably. The woman who had brought me there sprang forward with her hands outstretched. I recoiled with embarrassment. Hospital I was at home in, but home nursing was a thing I had to get used to. There had been an intimacy about the death upstairs that was less intrusive behind closed screens on a hospital ward. The shadows cast by the candle had troubled me greatly; the wind whistling down the wide old chimney had shaken me like a leaf.

'We're so grateful to you, dear, for all you've done for Grandma,' said the woman trying furtively to stuff a note into my hand. I let the note fall and it fluttered to the ground and came to rest between our feet. The thought of being offered money for the service I had rendered brought back the image of the intoxicated Mrs Gamp. I had never before been offered a tip. Even the millionaire I had once nursed through an attack of gout hadn't thought of rewarding me for being so kind to his big toe. Anything in the nature of a gratuity had been frowned upon in the days when I did my training. If a sister caught us accepting so much as a grape from a patient in return for all we had done for him, we could be in the Matron's office the next morning threatened with instant dismissal if we were ever caught in the act again.

I stood for a moment trying to think of a way of refusing the gift without offending the donor. At last I stooped down, picked up the note and handed it to the woman. 'Not at all,' I murmured softly. 'It's been a pleasure I'm sure.'

From the look on her face I knew at once that I had said the wrong thing. I blushed hotly, gathered the hem of my nightdress into the tops of my wellington boots and escaped through the door.

As I waded home through the puddles I thought of all the things I could have said that would have been more appropriate under the circumstances and reflected sadly that for people like me the right things to say are often only thought of long after the moment for saying them is past.

There had been many occasions when I failed to say the things that were expected of me, or failed to give answers that would satisfy the questioner. When the Roman Catholic lady from one of the houses opposite dropped in to see me one morning the nervous way she drank the tea I gave her told me that it wasn't just a social call. I could only hope that if it was a diagnosis she had come for the symptoms would be ones that I recognized. I had slipped up so often in putting a name to a complaint that I was rapidly losing confidence in myself as a diagnostician, and sometimes even losing confidence in myself as a nurse.

It was Dilys's mother who first alerted me to my waning powers. She had startled me one day in her kitchen by pulling her knickers down, her vest up and begging me to take a look at her abdomen. I searched for a long time among the pendulous folds but could find nothing worthy of a mention.

'What am I supposed to be looking for?' I asked at last, straightening my aching back.

'The scar, of course,' said Dilys's mother, stabbing at

a fold with her finger. I followed the moving finger until I came across a small indentation which I foolishly took to be the faded remains of a very old appendectomy.

'Why you clever old thing,' I cried admiringly. 'You've had your appendix out.'

She gave me a withering look. 'It wasn't me appendix, it was me chubes,' she said angrily.

I went hot with shame. There were times when I heartily wished that nobody had ever found out that I had once been a nurse. For a layman to confuse a single appendix with a whole set of tubes might be excusable, but for a nurse who is supposed to have spent years learning the difference it was unforgivable.

Dilys's mother forgave me and went on. 'They took the lot out at once,' she said pridefully. 'They said I'd be a new woman without them. And I was. Our Dilys was born nine months to the day after they did it. She was no bigger than a pound of sugar. They said she was a miracle.'

I agreed with whoever 'they' were. But whether I was agreeing because Dilys, who had started out as being no bigger than a pound of sugar, had made such a remark-able progress over the years, weighing in at not an ounce less than thirteen stones by the time she was sixteen, or because she had been conceived, carried and delivered without the aid of one solitary tube I couldn't be sure, so I forebore to comment on the miracle. Her another pulled down her vest, adjusted the rest of her dress and went home, clearly disgusted with me for not enthusing over her gynaecological history. Thinking about it later I could only assume that there had been some slight confusion with the dates. Dilys's mother was no longer young. Old ladies tend to grow forgetful and add or take away a year or two when they are describing the historical events in their lives. I do it myself sometimes and I am not yet old in the strictest sense of the word.

The Roman Catholic lady had not come to show me her abdomen. She sat nervously tying knots in the corner of my best chenille tablecloth.

'I hope you didn't mind me coming,' she said, raising her eyes and lowering them again quickly. 'I wondered if you could give me a bit of advice.'

I filled up her cup again hoping to distract her attention from the tablecloth. It had been a wedding present and I cherished it. There was a matching piece of chenille fringing nailed to the mantel shelf.

'What was it you wanted advice about?' I asked warily. I had learned from experience not to commit myself to offering advice until I had more of the facts. This saved embarrassment all round if I had no advice to offer.

'It's about the Pope,' said the woman, taking another tug at the tablecloth. I put the teapot back on the hob.

Being of the lowest possible denomination myself I knew very little about the Pope. I wasn't too informed about the Archbishop of Canterbury, and he was much closer to home than the Pope. 'You see,' the woman went on, 'I and my husband are Catholics and we have to do as the Pope tells us to do. We can't afford to have any more babies. The doctor I was under when I fell for the last one said he wouldn't be answerable for the consequences if it happened again. We only do it when the Pope says we can but we still seem to get babies. We wondered if you could tell us some way we could do it without going against the Pope.'

Sadly I couldn't. She went away no wiser than she was when she came and as disillusioned about people who had once been nurses as Dilys's mother was. Again I wished that nobody had discovered I was once a nurse.

While I was drinking what was left of the stewed tea I found myself marvelling that a man who kept himself to himself as much as the Pope was reputed to do should hold such sway over the love life of his flock. The way I saw it, the Roman Catholic lady could have as many more children as she had already got before natural processes took over, producing a method of birth control that would satisfy her, her husband and the Pope. Unless of course like Selina she started to put her foot down very firmly in bed. Or unless the doctor she was under at the time of her last conception had been right to disclaim responsibility for any that might follow.

Later that day I had another visitor. It was Davies, who had come to say goodbye to me. The goodbye saddened me. It was the end of an era for both of us.

Davies and I had done our training together and had worked together in the same hospitals while the war was on. It was only when I got married and left work a year later in the full flush of expectant motherhood that our lives had started taking a different course.

Davies had been engaged to a proud and aristocratic young man called Archibald almost from the start of the war. He had refused to marry her then. He could be killed, he said, and where would that leave Davies? It was a question that didn't have to be answered since he wasn't killed. Instead he lived so long behind bars in one of the worst prison camps that he might almost as well have been dead. The medal the King pinned on him after the war was over gave *The Times* plenty to comment on but was small compensation for all he had lost. Though his body had remained intact his pride was so severely wounded by the cruel spite of his jailers that he was a broken man.

When the war showed signs of coming to an end, Davies had taken the hand-embroidered huckaback towels out of her bottom drawer and started to plan her wedding outfit; but after she had seen what the prison camp had done to Archibald she put the towels back in their tissue paper and stopped thinking about a bridal gown. She knew her Archibald well enough to realize that if he had been unwilling to do anything as irresponsible as marrying her while he was a lusty young man he was hardly likely to contemplate such a drastic move now that he was so sadly defeated by the glorious victory.

So Davies was still Davies and still working at the Sanatorium we had gone to after we finished our training. Though she had visited me often the visits never quite recaptured the warmth of the friendship we had shared over the years when we had sat on each other's beds running down our seniors while we were still juniors, and picking on the juniors after we had become swollen-headed seniors. I was too caught up with the children and all the other things that marriage meant to me, and she saw too much that she would have liked for herself, and which it had begun to seem as if she would never have.

We sat for a while allowing the children to monopolize the conversation, then I bundled them out to play with promises of great treats later if they stayed outside while Auntie and I had a nice chat. They went reluctantly. Playing outside was something they could do any time; listening to Mummy and Auntie having a nice chat appealed to them far more than squabbling over a skipping rope or fighting to get possession of a doll.

As an opening to the conversation Davies showed me letters she'd had from Baker and Weldon. They had done their training with us and had been our closest friends for a long time. The last time I saw either of them had been on my wedding day when for a while it had seemed almost like old times again. But so much had happened since our training days that it was impossible for anything to be like old times again. Weldon's dream of having lots of babies for her soldier husband Harry to spoil when the war was over had ended abruptly when a bomb fell on his mother's house, killing Harry (who was home on leave at the time) and all his family but sparing Weldon who was on nights and had been refused a night off, even though her husband was home on leave, and it was more than a month since she'd had her last night off. Nights off in those days were more of a privilege than a right. They were seldom granted for something as unimportant as a husband having home leave. Being deprived of her night off had at least kept Weldon alive, but that was small comfort to her while she was watching them searching through the rubble for Harry and his family.

Baker, whom we had hoisted so often through her bedroom window when she came in later than the Matron's rules allowed, was never the same happy carefree girl after her sailor brother went down with his ship at the start of the war. The Irish doctor she married in a register office one morning with us all there as witnesses had managed to cling to the tail of his plane through night after night of savage attack, but he also had lost a lot of his youthful zest. So much had happened since our training days that it was better not to think too much about any of it.

I had suffered the least of any of us. I had the children that Weldon could only dream about through sleepless nights. I had a husband, which was something that Davies might never have, and I didn't have a brother drowned at sea. The war touched me very lightly.

After I had finished reading the letters Davies told me why she had come to see me.

'I've come to say goodbye,' she said. 'I'm leaving the Sanatorium.' I wasn't too surprised by her announcement. I had noticed signs of restlessness during her last two visits to me. She had complained more about the food in the sisters' dining room and had said sharper things about the patients than I had ever heard her say before. Saying sharp things about the patients had never been a habit with Davies. On the occasions that we had sat around in her bedroom discussing case histories she had always found an excuse for the patient who insisted he was ill when the doctors tried to tell him there was nothing wrong with him. Davies was always ready to see the patient's side. She quoted cases where the patient had come in complaining of nothing short of a ruptured appendix, and been assured that it was chronic constipation, only to be re-admitted a week later with something less than a ruptured appendix, but certainly more serious than constipation. She said it was never wise to disregard completely a patient's own diagnosis of his illness. I knew she was right. I too had nursed patients who came in protesting that all they were suffering from was a mild form of nettle rash. After extensive tests for diseases of which the rash could have been a symptom, the patients were sent home in disgrace, accused of wasting the doctor's time, not to mention taking up a hospital bed, when all that was wrong with them was a mild form of nettle rash. It wasn't always easy being a patient, unless the ward sister was as understanding as Davies had been before she started getting restless.

'Where are you going?' I asked her.

'I'm going back to our training school,' she said, surprising me at last. 'I saw an advertisement for a sister's post in the *Nursing Mirror*, and I answered it. The Matron accepted me. It's a new Matron now, you know. The old one died.'

I had heard through the hospital grapevine. I had found it hard to imagine the hospital without her and the fat Scottie dog that had bared his teeth and snarled at us whenever we went to the office in disgrace. He had bared his teeth and snarled at us whenever we went to the office, but he put more venom into the snarl when we were in disgrace. He could smell our fear, which was not surprising; we could smell it ourselves, pouring from our armpits and oozing from our sticky hands.

'Why did you decide to go back there?' I asked Davies, already knowing the answer before I asked the question. We had done our training in Nottingham, and Archibald lived there. If they were not to spend their life together, it was still important that they should see as much of each other as possible. Davies had spent all her days off since the war ended setting out with excitement at the prospect of seeing him and coming back saddened by the hopelessness of it all.

'It's Archibald,' she said. 'He lives with his aunts like he did before the war, and they aren't getting any younger. It'll make it easier for them and nice for him to have me around when they need me.' She smiled, looking for a moment more like the Davies I had known and been so fond of over many years.

'And when he's well again we shall be married and the children will be bridesmaids and you can be my matron of honour and hold the bouquet for me.' She stopped and I could see that she was thinking of the day when she had been my bridesmaid and had trailed up the aisle behind me wearing my second best pair of shoes that were two sizes too big for her. I didn't want her to see me crying, so I turned my head away.

When it was time for her to get back to the Sanatorium, I walked with her as far as the bus stop and then went home again. I called the children in from play and gave them a biscuit by way of an apology for being so snappy with them when Auntie was there. Suddenly I felt there was a great deal that I should be thankful for.

After Davies left the Sanatorium I thought about her often for a few weeks, then put her aside to find room in my thoughts for other things, the most absorbing being how we were going to pay the electricity bill when there was never enough money to keep the coalman happy. It was a problem that kept me awake for long hours during many nights. The solution to it was to set the pattern of our lives for the next few years: I went back to hospital and became a part-time nurse.

Chapter Four

THE TIDE IN our already muddled affairs had taken a turn for the worse the day the coal bill and the electricity bill fell on our mat with a combined plop just after we had spent our life savings on shoes and winter coats for the children. The cost of the combined plop ran almost into double figures. We were stupefied. Short of taking back the shoes and coats and fighting for a refund there seemed no way out of the deep financial waters we had squandered ourselves into. We went over the housekeeping bills penny by penny, weighing the necessity for this against the luxury of that and adding the cost of a gallon of paraffin for the oil stove to the price of a pint of methylated spirit for the primus stove. Both pieces of equipment were necessary where we lived. The primus stove was indispensable for making a quick cup of tea whenever the kitchen fire glowered blackly instead of glowing brightly enough to boil a kettle, and the oil stove was a standby for when the miners came out on strike as they so often did in the middle of an icy winter.

We didn't have an automatic cooker; neither did we have a car, a telephone or holidays on the Costa Brava. Cars and telephones were only just starting to come within reach of the masses and holidays on the Costa Brava were to be for the richer than us for a long time. The reason we didn't have a cooker was because there wasn't one in the house when we moved there and whenever we talked about buying one there was always something we were more urgently in need of. The oven, which relied on the heat from the glowing coals to get it in the mood for cooking, remained in active service until the day we went to live in another house where an automatic cooker headed the list of priorities.

At the end of all our adding and subtracting and tedious manipulation of the household accounts we had to face the grim reality that we would have been bankrupt but for the fact that we had never had any money in the bank. I prayed long and earnestly for something to turn up, and when it didn't I did what all the other women in the terrace did when they needed advice. I went to Selina.

The advice she gave me was short and startling. 'You'll have to get a job and go out to work,' she said, making it sound ridiculously easy.

Getting a job and going out to work was the very last

thing I would have thought of doing as a way of solving our problems. Though both the children had overcome an inherited reluctance to go to school and had even resigned themselves to eating their dinner under the watchful eye of a teacher, I could still find plenty to keep me busy at home. Almost every morning I swept a mat, dusted a chair and did the hundred and one other things that were the scheduled duties of a wife and mother. In the afternoon I pottered about in the garden and brought in the eggs that the pullets had kindly laid for us. If there was an egg left over after our daily needs were assessed I wiped it over with a damp cloth and placed it in a jar of isinglass to preserve it, not for posterity, but for the lean days when the pullets were moulting and stopped laying. Then I strolled to the school and stood at the gates waiting for the children to tumble out. My days were full. I hadn't a minute to spare for going out to work.

'I couldn't possibly get a job and go out to work,' I said to Selina.

'Why ever not?' she asked. I explained about sweeping the mat in the morning and preserving the egg in the afternoon and all the other things that kept me ungainfully occupied from morning to night. Her answer to this was brief. 'Rubbish,' she said.

I tried again, this time approaching it from a different angle.

'Look at it from a different angle,' I said. 'Think of the children. They need a mother.' My eyes moistened at the thought.

'They've got a mother,' Selina reminded me.

The truth of the statement and the blunt way it was made dried my eyes. But they wouldn't have, I said, if I got a job and went out to work. Where, I asked, would they be without me standing fresh as a daisy in the morning waving them into school, and waiting fresh as a daisy to welcome them out of it again in the afternoon? Selina gave the question a moment's thought before she answered it. The answer was as devoid of sentiment as all her other answers had been.

'Well, forgetting the fact that you're never as fresh as a daisy in the morning anyway I expect they'd be in my house after you'd gone to work until it was time for me to take them to school, and watching Muffin the Mule or Andy Pandy on our telly in the afternoon until you got back from work and collected them.' She had an answer for everything. She was also the first in the terrace to have a television set. Everybody had watched from their windows when the van pulled up and two men lifted out a twelve-inch console model, with doors that folded back when the picture was on, and carried it into Selina's house. It had caused a lot of gossip.

'Well, all I can say is good luck to them,' said Dilys's

mother. 'But you wait till we get a thunderstorm. I've heard that them aerials attract lightning quicker than anything.' After that whenever she thought she heard thunder in the distance she rushed out in breathless anticipation of Selina's house going up in flames. When it didn't she went inside again looking very upset.

Edna had been particularly bitter. She was bitter about most things; she had had a lot to make her bitter.

'What I'd like to know is where they get the money from,' she said, staring malevolently up at the aerial. 'Things like television sets don't get given away with tea coupons. It fell off the back of a lorry, I shouldn't wonder.'

It was only when the Coronation was imminent that Selina got back into favour with her neighbours. Then we all rushed out to rent a set and there were aerials springing up from every chimney and not a child to be seen playing in the garden when Andy Pandy was on.

After Selina had finished outlining her plans for standing in as a grandma to the children while I went out to work, I looked for other reasons why I should stay at home.

'My husband wouldn't like it,' I said, clutching at straws. 'He's got old-fashioned ideas about women going out to work. He says it's a man's job to support his family.' Though I had never actually heard him say such a thing I had no doubt that he would if the matter ever arose.

Selina gave a cynical snort. 'I shouldn't worry too much about that,' she said. 'He might surprise you. It's the same as I've always said about men: most of them will agree to anything if it's in their interest to agree and if you go the right way about making them agree. You just come straight out with it tonight and tell him you're going to get a job and go out to work, never mind what he cares to say about it.' Not for the first time I envied Selina her direct approach to life and its problems.

I waited until the children were in bed that night, then I came straight out with it and told my husband that I was going to get a job and go out to work, never mind what he cared to say about it. I didn't put it quite as bluntly as that and after I had finished going round in circles and beating about the bush he gave me a funny look.

'Are you trying to tell me you're going to get a job and go out to work?' he asked. I nodded and stood back an inch or two waiting for the storm. There was no storm. Instead a look of relief came over his face.

'Good idea,' he said, shovelling the bills back into the sideboard drawer. 'When are you going to start?' I felt sadly let down. I had expected to have to beg and entreat him before he lowered his pride enough to consent to me going out to work. I hadn't expected immediate capitulation or even the look of relief.

'Well, what did he say when you told him you were going to get a job?' said Selina when I saw her the next day. I took a deep breath and looked her straight between the eyes.

'He was furious,' I told her. 'Absolutely livid. He stormed and raved and went on for hours about it being a man's job to support his family. He only started to come round a bit when I told him that you'd offered to look after the children when he wasn't there and I was at work. Even then he wasn't too keen on the idea.' I hoped she would swallow the lies. She did.

'There, what did I tell you,' she said. 'Men are all the same.' I had to admit she was right.

Getting a job wasn't as easy as Selina had made it sound. The people whose 'situations vacant' advertisements I answered were always expecting me to do things I wasn't capable of doing. I had to be honest when the man behind the desk in the office asked me whether I could type: I couldn't do shorthand either. I disappointed the manageress of a canteen when, after all her cross-examination, she discovered that I had never cooked for numbers. I was hopeless when it came to balancing plates in a restaurant and my arithmetic was a stumbling block behind every shop counter. When the final demands started coming in and the bills became more pressing I went back to Selina. Again she had the solution.

'Why don't you try the factory down the road?' she said, after I had finished telling her of my lack of success in other fields. 'They wouldn't expect you to know anything there. You could start from scratch and work your way up. I should think even you could manage that.'

I doubted it and so did the man who interviewed me at the factory down the road. He didn't share her faith in my ability to adapt myself to a whole new way of life and learn a whole new set of skills.

'You'd never do it,' he said, looking me up and down in a slightly contemptuous way. 'You've never worked in a factory before, have you?'

I admitted that I hadn't but promised to do my best to give satisfaction if only he'd give me the chance. The promise didn't melt his heart.

'Where do you work now?' he asked.

I told him that I didn't work, I was just a housewife. I had already discovered that being a housewife wasn't an occupation that counted as work. There was more to work than cooking, cleaning, washing, poultry rearing and child minding.

'What were you doing when you were working?' he then asked.

When I told him that I had been a nurse he looked me up and down again, picked up the telephone and asked somebody on the other end of the line whether the Chief Fire Officer would kindly step that way. For a moment I thought I was about to be recruited into the factory fire service, and with memories still fairly fresh in my mind of the fire-fighting drill we did during the war, I knew I would be no better at that than I was at any of the other jobs I had applied for.

The fire officer's name was Bill. He was a sturdily built man with silvering hair and brown eyes. After he had a few words with the man behind the desk, he turned to me.

'If you were a nurse, then why aren't you a nurse now?' he said sternly.

'Because I've got two children,' I said, shrinking a little at the sternness in his voice. 'I couldn't leave them from eight o'clock in the morning to eight o'clock at night, or eight o'clock at night to eight o'clock in the morning to go and work in a hospital.' He raised his eyebrows a little and laughed.

'But it isn't like that in hospitals any more,' he said. 'Not even for the full-time nurses, and you're a married woman with children. You could work whatever hours would suit you best.'

I looked for signs that he was joking. The idea of any nurse being able to work whatever hours would suit her best was too absurd to be taken seriously.

'I'm not joking,' said Bill. 'I know what I'm talking about. My wife's a nurse, she works part-time up at the hospital, and most of the nurses up there are part-timers. A lot of them have got children as young as yours. I should go home and write to the Matron if I were you. Ask her if you can go up and see her. She'll be only too glad to have you, they're crying out for nurses.'

I walked out of the factory in a daze. It had never occurred to me that I could possibly go back to nursing at least while the children were so young. Nursing as I knew it was a full-time occupation, with only an hour or two off during the day or night and a day or night off when it was convenient to the ward. Nevertheless I wrote to the Matron of the hospital on the other side of the town from the Sanatorium, asking her if I could go and see her.

The immediacy of her reply left me in no doubt that Bill the fire officer had indeed known what he was talking about. She said she had been delighted to receive my letter and could I possibly go and see her the following Monday to discuss my domestic circumstances and decide upon the hours I thought I would be able to work. The speed at which it was all happening took my breath away, especially when I remembered all the preliminaries that had to be gone through in the past before going to be a nurse reached even the first stage.

The Matron was as big a surprise to me as her letter had been. She greeted me warmly, pulled up a chair for me in front of her desk and started by asking me how the children were. I told her how they were, beginning with their birth weight and ending up with the fuss they'd made only that morning when there'd been no clean socks for them to wear for school. I spared her nothing.

She waited patiently until there was a gap in the monologue wide enough for her to get a word in edgeways, then she asked me where I had done my training, how long ago and what I had been doing since. After I had exhausted that topic she quite casually asked me what hours I thought it would be possible for me to work.

Although the fireman had prepared me for the question, I was still taken aback by it. When I had recovered a little I gave her a brief run-down of my household commitments, from the moment I got up in the morning to the time I went wearily up the stairs to bed. I told her about Selina and how she had said she would have the children for me if I got a job and went out to work, and in the middle of the telling I remembered that the kindly woman who was listening to me was a Matron. The thought dried up the flow and the Matron took the opportunity to ask me another question.

'And what will happen to the children during the school holidays?' she asked with a warm touch of concern for the children in her voice.

I didn't know. I hadn't got as far as thinking about the school holidays. I thought about them for a moment.

'I expect Selina will have them for me,' I said, feeling almost sure that she would.

The Matron smiled. It was the sort of smile that one woman gives to another and not the chilly facial movement I had learned to expect from the Matrons of old.

'Then we will leave the question of the school holidays for you to arrange with her and come to some agreement over your hours. Do you think you would be able to work nine to three-thirty from Monday to Friday?'

For a moment I couldn't think at all. I was stunned by the thought of a hospital being willing to employ a nurse for six hours a day and for only five days a week. However much we might have needed the money, there seemed something not quite right in being paid for so little labour. The Matron saw the bemusement on my face and hastened to set my mind at rest.

'If you think you could manage to fit the hours in with your other commitments we would be happy to employ you on those terms. Since the war there have been so many other careers for girls to choose from that the hospitals are being faced with an acute shortage of nurses. We rely very heavily on our part-timers.'

For the first time I began to understand why I was

being invited to work a mere thirty hours a week with no weekends. The choice of careers for a girl had been far more limited when I was a girl. If she was rich and beautiful she stayed at home and did a little flower arranging for her mother until a beautifully rich young man carried her off to his hundred acres to do his flower arranging for him. If she was neither rich nor beautiful but had managed to pass a scholarship that took her to the high school she almost inevitably became either a nurse or a teacher. I had become a nurse, though it was not of my choosing. My mother had done the choosing for me. In those days mothers knew best what was good for their daughters.

The Matron continued: 'Having to run the ward with so many part-time nurses puts a heavy burden on the full-time staff, but that is the price we have to pay if we want to keep our wards open. You may be sure that whatever hours you work will be appreciated.' I realized she was trying to tell me that I didn't have to feel guilty at being only a part-timer. I went home amazed at the amazing things that had happened to nursing since I was last a nurse.

My husband burst in from the office that evening eager to hear the news.

'Well, how did it go?' he asked, breathless with hurrying. I told him how it had gone, and then he asked the question that was closest to his heart. 'How much are they paying you?' It was only after he had asked the question that I remembered the money had never been mentioned. His face fell. He went gloomily through the bills while he was eating his supper.

The next morning a letter came from the hospital finance office, clearing up some of the mysteries that hadn't been touched upon during the interview. There was a contract for me to sign on the dotted line, and several numbered notes telling me that I would be entitled to meals whenever my duties covered a meal time, to uniform and the laundering thereof, to an annual holiday *pro rata* to the hours I worked and to Industrial Insurance if I was unlucky enough to break my neck or a limb in the execution of my duties.

There was a final and staggering note which told me that as a staff nurse, part-time and non-resident, my wages would be two shillings and twopence an hour. I found a pencil and a piece of paper and after I had multiplied two shillings and twopence by thirty several times and arrived each time at the sum of sixty-five shillings I did the sum yet again. Sixty-five shillings for thirty hours' work seemed much too good to be true.

My husband, who was better at arithmetic than I was, checked on the figures, found they were correct and then tossed the bills in the air. We were rich – or we would be when I got my first pay packet.

Part Two

Chapter Five

GETTING UP IN the morning was something that had never come easy to me. As a child, I had often wakened in the springtime and listened to my parents muttering over their breakfast downstairs while they waited for the dawn chorus to start. In the winter they were up long before the dawn, crashing about in the chilly light of an oil lamp and a couple of candles. They were firm believers in the maxim that early to bed and early to rise brought health, wealth and wisdom to its devotees. Health and wisdom maybe, but riches were harder to come by. I had lost whatever faith I might once have had in the maxim the moment I left home to be a nurse. When the call nurse came dashing into our bedrooms at six o'clock in the morning to remind us that it was six o'clock and breakfast was at half-past, I was one of the sluggards who turned over and went back to sleep after she had gone. I was also among those who threw themselves down at the breakfast table just as the healthy, wealthy and wise ones were filing out with smug looks on their faces, ready to report on duty on the dot of seven.

Getting up to go to work after I became a part-time nurse was even more of a hardship to me. There were times when I could have cheerfully hurled the alarm clock through the bedroom window and turned over for a lot more sleep.

The role of wife and mother had been enough to keep me spasmodically employed from morning to night; but with another role thrown in, the spasms of unemployment were reduced considerably. It was clear from the start that something would have to suffer and inevitably it was the housework that suffered. I was never addicted to housework: it was something I could always put off till tomorrow, if there was something more interesting to do today. Selina, who prided herself on being the most houseproud woman in the terrace, found it hard to understand how anybody could sit and read the papers before the beds were made. I regularly read the paper before I made the beds, but however much I tried to convince her that the daily news had an excitement that the daily bed making lacked she, who saved Andy Capp for her elevenses, was never convinced.

'Well, I suppose we can't all be alike, and far be it from me to criticize,' she would say, averting her critical eye from the dust on the sideboard. 'But I do like to get the beds made first. Supposing somebody was took bad in a hurry and the doctor came and found the bed not made?'

I refused to dwell on such a catastrophic possibility. I remembered my mother saying much the same sort of thing in much the same sort of voice when she had insisted on me changing my knickers before I walked up to the village to post a letter.

'Now you get them off and put these on,' she would say, standing over me while I removed the offending garment. 'What if something was to run over you with dirty knickers on while you were walking to the post office, I'd never be able to lift my head in church again.' Since nothing ever had run over me with dirty knickers on, I had become as fatalistic about it happening as I was about the doctor coming and finding the beds not made.

The first day that I went back to work the beds were made early enough to satisfy even Selina, the worst of the dust had been removed in the week after I went to see the Matron and, to the casual observer, the house had a semblance of cleanliness. The fanatic looking for cobwebs would not have been too disappointed. If Rome wasn't built in a day, then neither was the lived-in appearance of our house destroyed in a week.

The family's reaction to my new-found morning energy was perhaps only to be expected. They had grown accustomed to seeing me lolling over a frying pan or dozing over Quaker Oats. The children went into shock when I hinted at the top of my voice that the time had come for them to start doing up their own buttons and tying their own shoelaces. They developed a mental block which rendered them incapable of distinguishing left from right, inside from out and back from front. They reduced their IQs to zero and each of them became a helpless clinging little woman, which was something I had always wanted to be, but never seemed to get the technique right. Helpless I may often have been, but little I most certainly was not.

Their father took his cue from the children. He sat for a long time with an empty cup in front of him waiting for me to fill it. When I suggested with as much tolerance as I had time for that morning that a grown man might reasonably be expected to have mastered the art of pouring out a cup of tea, he reminded me with much the same degree of tolerance that it was a woman's job to pour out tea. I brought the discussion on equal rights to a head by issuing the ultimatum that he either poured or went without. He poured, but the atmosphere had grown very tense by the time he grouched off to work.

Taking the children round to Selina created more dissension. Despite the many hours they had spent in her house being plied with apples, sweets and sticky buns, they raised all sorts of objections to being dragged round there with egg stains still on their chins. (The egg stains were still on their chins because at the final five minutes nobody could find a face flannel.) We walked down the terrace to the accompaniment of sobs and sniffles from the youngest and a lot of muffled acrimony from her sister. I was silent but seething. I had reached the stage where whatever I had said would have been too much.

When Selina asked why the little loves looked so miserable that morning I said it was perhaps because I had been irritable with them, having lain awake most of the night worrying about leaving them with a neighbour – however kind the neighbour was – while I was gallivanting off to work. The kind neighbour drew the children towards her.

'You shouldn't have fretted over them,' she said, slapping a wet rag across the egg stains and giving them a final polish with a kitchen towel. 'It's as I've always said about children: they've got to learn to stand on their own feet sometime and the sooner they start learning the better.' She took the youngest on her lap, thereby ensuring that she didn't have to stand on her own feet while her tears were being dried and her nose blown.

When they were both at peace again Selina produced a stick of rock from the dresser drawer and shared it out between them. The rock was some she had brought back when she and Dilys's mother went to Southend for the day. They often went to Southend for the day. They said the mud did marvels for their feet. The rock did marvels for the children's morale. They were all smiles when I left them which made it easier for me to go.

At nine o'clock I reported to the Matron. She beamed when she saw me and said how nice it was that I had managed to get there on time. So many part-timers didn't, she said, especially those with children. Children were so apt to wake up crying with earache, or some other small complaint that was big enough to keep their mothers at home. She sounded as if it happened often enough not to surprise her any more.

She gave me five white coats trimmed with navy blue epaulettes, a navy blue belt and six curiously shaped pieces of starched white linen that had to be cunningly transformed into six curiously shaped starched white caps. Making them up gave me as much trouble as the butterfly caps that my fingers had fumbled over while I was a probationer nurse.

The Matron said she hoped the coats would fit me: they weren't new, but the nurse who had worn them last was roughly my size. By that I gathered that the nurse who had last worn them was amply built, with wide hips and full bosom.

She then asked me if I would mind going on to a female chronic ward for the time being. Though the sister there was always short of staff she was more than usually short of staff that morning. I said I didn't mind at all, which was true. In fact I welcomed the idea. I had no wish to be thrust into the hurly-burly of a busy acute ward on my first day back at work after a break of nearly ten years; a little light chronic nursing with no responsibilities would be a good start to my rehabilitation. I wouldn't have been as complacent if I could have foreseen the next few hours.

I walked across to the changing room that the Matron directed me to. The cold and cheerless room was empty except for a few odd shoes scattered around and a few cigarette ends that had been stubbed out on the floor. One of the tall green lockers that were obviously intended to be used as wardrobes by the part-time nurses already had my name slotted in the space provided, which with the scattered shoes and the stubbed-out cigarette ends gave me a warm feeling of being a nurse again, even if I was only a nurse in parts. I had already temporarily cast off the other two parts: the roles of wife and mother would be waiting for me when I got home again, but until then I was a nurse.

I was very disappointed in the uniform I had been given, despite the fact that the coats fitted me with an inch to spare all round. I had expected full regalia. Without the striped dress, the starched apron and the lacy bows of the bonnet I wore when I became a staff nurse there seemed nothing, except perhaps the navy blue belt and epaulettes, to tell anybody what I was. It brought back memories of the morning when Davies and I first went to work at the Sanatorium and a woman had brought us a cup of tea in bed. She had worn a white coat bedecked with epaulettes and Davies and I had immediately assumed that she was some sort of high-grade cook. She assured us loftily that she was not a cook but some special sort of wartime nurse, and we had to apologize very profusely to her. I hoped that nobody would mistake me for a cook.

The sister on the female chronic ward made no error of identification. She looked me up and down, took in the plainness of the ensemble I was wearing and groaned. The groan was one of deepest despair.

'Oh my God, not another part-timer,' she said. 'The Matron must be out of her mind. She knows I've only got one full-time student and a full-time assistant nurse.' Then, without waiting for me to apologize for being another part-timer she turned and hurried off. I hurried after her.

The ward we hurried into was quite small. At a quick glance round I counted twenty beds. Dotted among the beds were a number of elderly ladies sitting in armchairs. The ladies were wearing dresses or jumpers and skirts that had ceased to be fashionable a long time ago. At first I thought they were sitting patiently waiting for a porter to come and wheel them away somewhere, then I realized what had happened.

A long time ago an eager young doctor had arrived at my training school, full of bright ideas about the care of chronic patients. He had outlined a plan for getting them up and allowing them to sit in chairs instead of keeping them in bed from the moment they were admitted to the moment they died. He even suggested that they should be taken to the lavatory whenever they wanted to go. He said it would save a lot of bedsores and be a lot better for the patients than having to be in cot beds all the time.

Fortunately for the hard-pressed nurses who worked on the forty or fifty-bedded chronic wards, the sisters in charge of them came out strongly against the suggestion. They knew only too well what it would lead to if the headstrong young man was allowed to have his way: patients sitting about everywhere, cluttering up the wards, and nurses having to work even harder than they already did, getting people up in the morning and putting them back to bed at night, not to mention the trips to the lavatory.

The young man's enthusiasm for his plan soon died down in the teeth of the opposition he got from the sisters. They ruled their wards with an iron hand; they weren't likely to let a young upstart like him tell them how to nurse their patients.

He would have been very happy to see the ladies on this ward, sitting about in chairs wearing their outdated jumpers and skirts instead of lying in bed in their winceyette nightdresses. But a ward of twenty beds was easier to manage than forty or fifty jammed tightly together. For one thing, there was plenty of space for armchairs between the beds.

The sister stopped in her tracks. 'We'll take those who are already up out on to the verandah first,' she said, adjusting the frilly band round her rolled-up sleeve. She advanced on one of the chairs and the patient who was sitting on it shrank back in anticipation of what she had learned from experience was about to happen to her.

'Come on, Gran,' the sister bawled kindly into her deaf old ear. 'It's a lovely day and the sun's shining. We're going to take you out on to the verandah. You'll like it there – you'll be able to sit and look at the flowers.'

Gran scowled at me from under her wispy fringe of white hair. Even she knew that it was more permissible to scowl at a plain coat with only epaulettes to identify rank than at a sister's dull dress uniform.

'I don't want to sit on the verandah, and I don't want to look at no flowers,' she snorted angrily. 'I just want to be left in peace. I'm sick to death of you lot pushing me around. I'm thinking of getting on to the higher authorities and having it stopped.'

It took the sister several minutes to explain that she was the higher authority, then we led the old lady slowly up the ward and sat her down on a chair on the verandah overlooking a garden of flowers. There was also a nice view of distant fields, but she was in no mood for views. She was still muttering fiercely about getting on to the higher authorities after we had tucked blankets round her arthritic old knees and put enough pillows into the hollow of her back to make her admit at last that she was sitting comfortably. She admitted it in very grudging tones.

'I sometimes wonder if it's worth it,' the sister said as we were walking up the ward to fetch another reluctant patient to the verandah. 'We almost give ourselves hernias getting them up in the morning and putting them back to bed later on, as well as trotting them to the lavatory whenever they say they want to go, and hardly any of them appreciate it. I'm sure they'd be just as happy, or just as unhappy, if we let them stay in bed.' Her shoulders sagged a little with despondency, then she brightened up again. 'But it does stop them getting bedsores, and it must surely be nicer for them to sit looking at the flowers on the verandah than sitting in the ward all day looking at each other. Though you'd never think so sometimes if you saw how they glare at each other out there.'

We went on almost giving ourselves hernias until every patient who could put one foot in front of the other, and many of those who couldn't, were out on the verandah. A few of them stubbornly refused to look at the view. Admitting that they liked it would have put their seal of approval on the daily exercise, and they were determined not to give us the satisfaction of doing that.

Sally, who was nearly a hundred, was one of the last to submit angrily to being moved from one chair to another. Before she submitted she told me her reason for wanting to stay put instead of giving in gracefully.

'See here, young woman,' she said, pounding her stick on the floor to accentuate each word. 'I'm nearly a hundred and I've worked hard all my life. All I'm asking is to be allowed to spend the little that's left of it lying quietly in my bed. Surely that's not too much to ask.'

I realized that living to be nearly a hundred must have been very wearing for her, and I was almost tempted to agree that it would be kinder to leave her to lie comfortably in her bed, then I thought of the days when she would have had no choice but to stay in bed, with flower gardens but a dim memory and a visit to the lavatory a forgotten luxury. I wheeled her out to the verandah and wrapped her in shawls. Then I looked back and saw her sitting glaring ferociously at the lady in the next chair. When she saw me looking back at her she glared ferociously at me instead. I gave her a little wave which infuriated her more and made her toss her head in anger. Then I went back into the ward.

'We'll do Jennie next,' said the sister, looking at her watch. 'Then it will be time for us to go into the kitchen and have our coffee. That's if Lottie has remembered to make the coffee. She's the domestic. She's an awful old hag but we put up with her.' From the affectionate way she spoke about Lottie I gathered she was loved by all.

Jennie was very young. Perhaps no more than twenty. She had bright searching eyes that took in the navy blue epaulettes and made her look questioningly at the sister. Her contracted limbs and tightly clenched hands told their own story. Something that had probably started off as being nothing much to worry about when she was a child had progressed rapidly until it had become a crippling disease that held no future for Jennie except years of lying in chronic wards surrounded by patients old enough to be her grandmother – unless something happened to shorten her life expectation.

The sister told her that I was the new part-time staff nurse, and Jennie laughed gleefully at the thought of the Matron sending me when the sister wanted a full-time nurse. It didn't take much to make Jennie laugh. She even laughed when we almost dropped her as we were lifting her out of bed. Though she was only a tiny curled-up ball, it wasn't easy to get a good grip of her. She didn't make it any easier for us by shaking violently whenever we seemed to be in control. But at last she was in the wheelchair and on the verandah. The sister chose a spot for her where she could see across the fields and into the flower garden, and she sat drinking in the beauty of the flowers as if storing it up for the long winter days that lay ahead of her.

After we had rushed one or two patients to the lavatory only to discover that they were false alarms we washed our hands and went to the kitchen. I was limping badly. The concentrated effort of the past hour or two had already taken its toll of my feet, grown tender with the easy living they had had since the last time they'd walked me up a ward in uniform. They would need plenty of soaking in salt water before they were in a fit state to get me through a day without torture. I would also need to spend part of my first pay packet on a pair of comfortable shoes. The Matrons of old had known what they were doing when they included two pairs of comfortable house shoes on the list of requirements they sent to our mothers before we went off to be nurses. I could have done with just one pair of comfortable house shoes on that first day back at work: latent corns leapt to life and seats of inflammation throbbed and burned. My feet were killing me, but it was a slow and painful death.

The woman in the kitchen, who was obviously Lottie, was little and thin and looked much too old to be still at work. She had a knot of faded red hair from which hairpins stuck out like porcupine quills. They fell about the floor whenever she made a point of shaking her head. A cigarette hung almost permanently from the corner of her mouth, making her do whatever she happened to be doing at any given moment with her eyes half closed to protect them from the smoke that curled up from the smouldering cigarette. She had no teeth.

She was busy burning toast when we went into the kitchen. The sister took a double saucepan off the kitchen stove and poured two cups of steaming coffee from it.

'Hurry up, Lottie, and get the toast scraped, we haven't got all day,' she said sharply.

Lottie ignored her and went on scraping the burnt toast over the sink until whatever whiteness there was about the sink was liberally speckled with black crumbs. She smeared two slices of the scraped bread with marg and slapped them down in front of us, then stood and watched us while we ate them. Or rather, she stood and watched me. She had seen the sister before but I was new. She regarded me from all angles; then, as if not too sure what conclusions to come to about me, she gave me a final long stare and started slamming cups on to a trolley ready for the patients' mid-morning drinks. I was glad to escape her scrutiny, but I was still inhibited about eating the toast. In the past eating in the kitchen was as sinful as accepting a grape from a patient. If we occasionally transgressed by doing either it was a matter between ourselves and our own conscience, or between us and whichever of our seniors caught us sinning.

But I was too hungry to stay inhibited for long. The alarm clock had been set to go off so early and I had eaten my Quaker Oats so long ago that I was ravenous. I quelled whatever guilt feelings I had and got on with my elevenses.

While we were gobbling the toast and gulping down the scalding coffee I got the answers to some of the questions I had been dying to ask since the moment I reported on duty that morning: the most perplexing being why I was the only nurse on duty, and why the sister was having to work like a junior instead of sitting in her office doing only the things that were expected of somebody of such high rank. All the sisters I had worked for before had been there for the sole purpose of seeing that their wards were in perfect shape when the Matron or the doctors did their daily rounds. They cracked the whip to keep their nurses on their toes and meted out off-duty as the whim took them. Only under the most exceptional circumstances had they rolled up their sleeves and become one of the workers. But this sister had slaved as hard as I had slaved. She had even hurried to the sluice to fetch a bedpan when an urgent cry rose from somebody who was too ill to be moved from her bed. The sight of a sister giving out a bedpan had caused me considerable embarrassment until I grew more accustomed to it. I had to tell myself that the reason she got to the sluice before me was because her feet were in better condition and she was thinner than I was and could hurry faster. She was tall and slim and very nice to look at. With all her visible assets I was surprised to see that there was no ring of any sort on her fourth finger. I was to learn later that she was a born nurse and wanted no other life for herself than the one she had.

'We are the only ones on until after first lunch,' she said, talking with her mouth full and shouting to make herself heard above the clatter that Lottie was making with the crockery. 'That's the reason we're having our coffee break on the ward. It's only allowed when there isn't enough staff on duty to keep the ward covered. At least we'd get a bit of peace in the dining room instead of having to be deafened by the domestic throwing the cups about.' She glared at Lottie, who answered by dropping a saucer on the floor. 'There should have been an auxiliary on with us this morning, but she rang to say that her little boy's got measles and she will have to do a late shift to give her mother time to get over and look after him while she's at work. He goes to the nursery school when he hasn't got measles. I'd already told the student nurses they could have the morning off and they don't like having their off-duty changed at the last minute. So it left just the two of us on.'

As I listened I tried to adjust to a situation where nurses didn't come on duty because their little boy had measles, and where student nurses took their off-duty whether they could be spared or not, simply because they didn't like it to be changed at the last minute. I thought of all the off-duty I had been robbed of over the years because the ward sister had decided in her wisdom that I couldn't be spared, and all the meals I had missed by being in the bathroom polishing taps when I should have been at lunch, tea or supper. I realized glumly that times had changed too late for me and all the other nurses who were probationers in the days when polishing the bathroom taps had priority over meals.

The sister poured out another cup of coffee for us both and went on to tell me enough about her staffing problems to explain the cool reception she had given me when I reported on duty that morning. That I was a staff nurse, wearing a navy blue belt and navy blue epaulettes, didn't altogether compensate for my being yet another part-timer. She would perhaps have been happier with a full-time nurse of whatever rank. A first-year student would at least not have thrown the ward into confusion by ringing up to say that one of her children was suffering from the plague that was currently emptying the schools and that she wouldn't be in until the quarantine period was over. I began to feel very sorry for the sister. Although my own young children had obligingly got over measles, chicken pox and whooping cough before I started back to work I knew only too well that there were still one or two surprises they could spring on me that would make it necessary for me to stay at home.

We finished off the toast and drained the coffee cups, and then hurried back into the ward. I went down to the verandah to make sure that nothing dire had befallen anybody while we were in the kitchen. It all looked exactly the same as it did when we left it, but despite the friendly grouping of the chairs that the sister had tried so hard to achieve, not one of the old ladies was having a nice little chat with the old lady next to her. They very rarely did. The friendly grouping was never the beginning of a lasting friendship. The chairs were pushed and shoved with walking sticks until the groups were rearranged into two opposing lines of cold enmity.

Sally, who was nearly a hundred, was an expert at splitting up groups. If she happened to be the first to get taken to the verandah, she surveyed the grouping with an evil eye, then proceeded to make wide sweeps with the end of her stick until each chair stood in splendid isolation from the others. If we were very busy and had no time to spare for reforming the groups, the patients sat all day with their backs to each other, often staring at a wall. None of them ever complained; they seemed to prefer it that way.

Sally was an expert at doing other things that annoyed people. She pushed windows open with her ferrule, or asked for them to be opened when all around were begging for them to be shut; and she shut them with a bang when the majority had voted for them to be opened. She became more garrulous than the Ancient Mariner when a little hush was called for, and pursed her mouth into an obstinate line when the doctor asked her urgent questions about her bowels. She was a typical example of a sweet old lady who has grown too old to be sweet. She got a great deal more satisfaction from being stubborn.

I stood for a moment looking at the patients. The morning sun had soothed some of them into a gentle doze, while others were huddled in their own thoughts, looking rapt but maybe thinking what they would be having for dinner that day. Only Jennie's eyes lit up when she saw me. I tucked her back into her blankets and tightened a safety strap to stop her slipping out of them again. Then I said something to make her laugh and walked away from her. I had forgotten how to remain detached about girls like Jennie. The chronic sick who have already grown old are easier to bear than the chronic sick as young as she was; they are less of a drain on the emotions. I knew that being a nurse I shouldn't have such emotions, but I was after all only a nurse in parts.

For the rest of that morning the sister and I did the things that had to be done. We ignored the cups that cluttered the lockers but we watched over Ella while she had one of her epileptic attacks. We left the linen unsorted to find time to do one or two of the daily baths before the lunches came up. We were both in the bathroom when the Matron arrived to do her round. Neither of us realized she was there until she spoke. The granny we were trying to coax into the bath was refusing to put her leg over the side.

'All this new-fangled bathing,' she grumbled crossly. 'It does nothing but weaken the spine.'

'The sooner you get in the sooner you'll be out, then your spine won't have time to weaken,' said the sister, urging the old lady to lift a leg. We had just managed to persuade her to dabble the toes of one foot in the water when the Matron said 'Good morning.'

Swiftly, the granny removed her toes from the water.

'Thank goodness you've come,' she said. 'I hope you can knock some sense into these two. Bathing me every day – I keep telling them it weakens the spine but they won't listen to me.'

The Matron stepped across, smiled kindly at the old lady and with one neat movement from the three of us the granny went into the bath with a very small splash.

She was so surprised at suddenly finding herself wallowing in warm water that she was reduced to silence long enough for the Matron to exchange a word or two with the sister about the staff situation, a few more about the rest of the patients and one or two with me about my first day back at work before she went on her way, presumably to finish the round.

I fished the soap from somewhere under the granny's bottom, the sister found the sponge and we got on with the bathing.

'Doesn't the Matron mind having to do the round without you?' I asked, lifting my voice above a fresh outbreak of complaints from the old lady: the water was too cold, too hot, there wasn't enough of it, there was too much of it, her spine was getting weaker all the time.

'She doesn't have to mind,' called back the sister. 'She knows we're always desperately short of staff, and she understands that I can't just drop everything to walk round the ward with her. Although I nearly dropped the patient when I realized she was standing in the bath-room.'

We dried the patient, dredged her with talcum powder and took her, still complaining, back to the verandah. We went through the routine so often that, by the time the porter appeared on the ward with the dinner trolley, I had started to rue the day when somebody had finally decided that chronic patients would benefit by being got up instead of being allowed to stay in bed, and would enjoy having a proper bath instead of being washed down in bed between two blankets. Whatever the advantages it might have had for the patients there were one or two disadvantages for the nurses, especially for those who had been out of practice for as long as I had. My feet, legs and back ached as they hadn't ached since the day I started my training. I felt ten years older than when I reported on duty that morning. I hoped the ageing process wasn't progressive. At the rate it was creeping up on me I would be in one of the cot beds myself by the end of the week.

When we started to give out the dinners, Lottie abandoned her polishing rags and scouring powders and came to help us. This shocked me very much at first. A domestic giving out the dinners was as bad or worse than a sister giving out the bedpans. It went against the order of things. A sister was for sitting in her office thinking up ways of thwarting her nurses, a domestic was for dropping saucers in the kitchen. I had to remind myself that racing round the ward with plates full of stew or dishes of rice pudding could hardly be described as a highly skilled nursing procedure before I could properly appreciate the help that Lottie gave us. She didn't just race round with plates and dishes, she nagged the naggers into accepting the food she offered them instead of demanding impossible luxuries like properly cooked rice pudding or gravy with no globules of grease floating on the top. She fed the helpless, obligingly blowing on their stew to cool it, and she screamed loving curses at Jennie when she shook so much that as much of her dinner fell into her lap as went down her throat. And when the last drop of rice pudding had been scraped up and the last plate collected in, she fell on to a chair in the kitchen and lit a cigarette.

'Gawd, I needed that,' she said, inhaling deeply.

I knew how she felt. I too had needed the comfort of nicotine when the stresses of life became too much for me, until the strain of morning sickness took away the craving. When the morning sickness went and the craving returned I appeased it with enormous quantities of extra-strong peppermints. Soon I was having to find something to appease the craving for extra-strong pepper-mints. In the end, there was nothing but willpower for me to fall back on. It wasn't as nice as nicotine but would do me far less harm or so the experts were just beginning to tell us, though it wasn't fear that forced me to give up smoking, it was inflation.

At one o'clock, the student nurse reported on duty. I was somewhat surprised when I saw her. The sister hadn't thought it worth mentioning that she was a beautiful brown-skinned girl who later told me that she came from the West Indies. The sister hadn't thought it worth mentioning because when another pair of hands is urgently needed all that matters is that the hands are gentle and kind, especially if they belong to a nurse. I was very impressed when the student nurse told me she came from the West Indies. I had never met anybody from there before. I wasn't even sure if I'd know where to look for them on the map. But later when I went across to the dining room for my lunch I was surprised again at the number of brown-skinned girls sitting at the tables. I hadn't known that the news of the plight our hospitals were in had spread across the world, bringing a bevy of eager immigrant girls to the rescue.

I ate the lunch, which tasted no different from all the other hospital lunches I had eaten over the years. Then I went back to the ward fortified, I hoped, against whatever shocks and surprises the afternoon would bring. I was being over-optimistic. It would have taken more than a hospital lunch to give me the strength I needed to sustain me until three-thirty.

Chapter Six

THE TIME I spent with the sister in her office after I got back from lunch might almost have been spent in my sitting room at home. The atmosphere was so relaxed and friendly that for a moment I was tempted to kick my shoes off under the chair to bring a little relief to my aching feet. But I quickly resisted the temptation. Despite the permissiveness that had crept into hospital discipline over the years, I was still old-fashioned enough to feel there had to be a line drawn somewhere in deference to one so senior to me. I kept the shoes on and suffered the torment of my feet in brave silence.

Lottie shuffled into the office with three cups and an old aluminium teapot full of coffee and hovered expectantly while the sister poured. The third cup had obviously been intended as a hint. When she saw that nobody was going to take the hint, she shuffled out again and returned almost at once with an assortment of tools for her trade. Though she didn't say a word, the black cloud on her face told us that, if she wasn't to be invited to have coffee with us, she would make it her business to see that we didn't enjoy ours. She swept the floor under our feet, polished the chair under our bottoms and cleaned around us with so much venom that it was quite impossible to make ourselves heard above the noise she was making. In answer to the sister's bawled request that she should go away and clean somewhere else until we had finished talking, Lottie reminded her that it was Monday, and Monday was her day for turning out the office come what may. It was only after she had drunk the coffee she black-mailed the sister into giving her that she remembered with innocent surprise that Monday was her day for washing the light bulbs in the ward and not for turning out the office as she had foolishly thought – silly old her. She collected up her tools and left us in peace.

The sister had taken me into her office to tell me a few things she thought I should know about the ward and its patients, and also to remind me that I would be in charge after she went off duty for the afternoon until I also went off duty at three-thirty.

The thought of being left in charge of a ward for even so short a time sent the coffee swirling around inside me. I wasn't prepared for so much responsibility so soon. I needed time to rid myself of the shackles of domesticity and become a fully paid-up member of the nursing profession again. I knew only too well that, because I was State Registered, everybody would expect me to know everything. I didn't know everything. There had never been a time in the whole of my nursing career when I had known everything, and with so many years doing other things than nursing much of what I had once known could only be dimly recalled. I also knew from the various nursing journals that I had scraped up enough coppers to buy, or had glanced through in the library, that there were a great many things being done in hospitals these days and a great many different ways of doing them of which I had no practical experience. Reading about them in the library was no sure way of learning how to do them. Coming back to be a part-time nurse would almost be like starting my training again. As with points of law, pleading ignorance would be no excuse if I failed to do the right thing. I could already see great chasms of ignorance yawning at my feet.

As well as reminding me of the responsibility that I was about to have to shoulder, the sister reminded me that the doctor still hadn't done his round. This struck chill in my heart. The memory of the pomp and ceremony of the doctors' rounds in the past filled me with forebodings for the one that loomed before me in the future. I was glad I had emptied the coffee cup. I knew I wouldn't have been able to hold it steady between my trembling fingers.

The sister recognized the signs of panic and did her best to reassure me. She was obviously used to having day-old part-time staff nurses who had been wives and mothers for so long that their fingers shook at the thought of doing anything more in the way of nursing than putting a plaster on a grazed knee.

'There's nothing you need to worry about,' she lied kindly, seeing me worrying. 'There'll be one or two chests for him to go over and some blood to be taken from bed number twenty.'

The casual way she threw in the bit about the blood made my own blood run cold. Going over one or two chests I could cope with. It would merely be a matter of baring one or two bosoms and keeping woolly vests and any other garments the patients might be wearing well out of the way of the stethoscope. It wasn't necessary to be a State Registered nurse to make a success of that. But taking blood from bed number twenty was a different matter altogether. In the first place it would require a tray to be got ready. I hadn't laid up anything more complicated than a tea tray since I left hospital, and even on that I had been known to omit something vital: a milk jug, a sugar basin, or even, on occasions, the teapot.

I did a quick run-through in my head of the things I thought the doctor might need. There seemed to be no great gaps in my memory but, bearing in mind the articles and the advertisements I had read in the nursing journals, I knew there could be a dozen things the doctor might ask for that I wouldn't recognize if I saw them. I trembled afresh. Again the sister did her best for me.

'If you should get stuck with anything and need help, you can always ask the assistant nurse who comes on at two. She's quite a character, but you'll like her. She was up at the Sanatorium before she came here. She should have taken her finals but things happened at home so she never got the chance. But because of all the experience she'd had they let her go on the Assistant Nurses' Roll without doing any special training for it. She's a marvellous nurse; she could run the ward as well as any sister.'

I wasn't completely happy at the sister's assessment of the assistant nurse's capabilities. Whether I liked her or not didn't make me any more anxious to turn to her for help. Having to show my ignorance to the ignorant would be painful enough, but having to reveal it to the more knowledgeable – and she an assistant nurse who should have taken her finals and could run a ward as well as a sister – would be a very humiliating thing for me to do. I prayed that the need would never arise.

At two o'clock the sister went off duty and two women reported on. One of them wore a coat even plainer than mine, with not an epaulette anywhere about it. I guessed at once that she was the auxiliary whose little boy had so disrupted the ward by having the measles. I tried not to feel too strongly against him for my aching muscles and throbbing feet.

The other woman was older and wore a white coat with pale blue epaulettes. I knew her well: her name was Brown. We had worked together at the Sanatorium! It was she who had lent me her broken-down old bicycle to ride from the ward to the dining room when we were on nights together and had so ably come to the rescue whenever I needed rescuing on those busy wartime nights. She had also rolled up her sleeves threateningly and downed a couple of pints before sorting out a crowd of gate-crashing evacuees who were having a knees-up in the house where I was lodging at the time. She had charged in, taken control of the situation and put everybody in their proper places with absolutely no fuss at all. I had a tremendous respect for Brown. If an emergency arose when I needed help there was nobody I would rather turn to than her.

We looked at each other and she was the first to speak. Being the phlegmatic sort of woman she was, it would have taken more than my unexpected appearance on the ward to throw her into a fever of excitement.

'Well, fancy seeing you here,' she said, showing as much enthusiasm as she felt the occasion merited. 'I must say, you've put on a bit of weight since I saw you last. Marriage must have agreed with you.'

It was just the sort of greeting I would have expected to get from her. She had never been one to suck up to her seniors by making flowery speeches.

'I bet Sister wasn't too happy at getting another part-timer,' she went on. 'She'd hoped for a full-timer to make up for the one that left last week.' I felt very cast down at being such a tremendous disappointment to everybody, but since there was nothing I could do about it, I realized it would be a waste of time trying to defend my honour as a part-time staff nurse.

When the preliminaries had been said and I had recovered from the shock of being confronted by Brown, I gave her a brief resume of all the things that had happened to me since the last time I saw her, using the children as my excuse for the extra poundage. She listened, only interrupting occasionally to throw in one or two rude comments that would have sounded much ruder if they had been thrown in by anybody but Brown. She had always had the happy knack of being able to make the most outrageous utterance sound as innocent as a quote from the Bible, unlike a nurse I once knew who only had to say 'Damn you' in the sweetest possible way to make whoever she said it to shrink back as if they could already feel the flames of hellfire licking round their heels.

After I had exhausted the story of my life, Brown gave me a brief outline of hers, and then it was the turn of the auxiliary nurse to introduce herself to me. She told me her name was Lynch, leaving me in no doubt at all that she was one of the Irish Lynches. She filled us in on every spot of her boy's little measles. When she finally arrived at the harrowing scene where she had had to tear herself away from him and leave him in the tender care of his grandmother, Brown looked round the ward.

'Where's Bailey?' she asked. Bailey was the girl who had so impressed me by telling me she came from the West Indies. I hadn't seen her since she reported back after second lunch. She had missed all the thrills of my children's chicken pox, measles and whooping cough, and had escaped Lynch's little boy's measles.

'She's on the verandah talking to Jennie,' said Lottie who had missed nothing. Whenever there was a bit of idle chat going on in the ward Lottie could be relied upon to be there, broom resting firmly on the floor while she rested firmly on the broom. No conversation piece would have been complete without Lottie forming part of it, her head nodding in agreement or shaking in violent dissent, sending hairpins spinning to the floor and the cigarette bobbing up and down from the corner of her mouth. 'I reckon it's a shame a young girl like Jennie having to be in a ward like this. I reckon there should be proper places for them to go to, not stuck in here with all these old grannies.' I remembered thinking along the same lines myself when we were taking Jennie to the verandah.

Brown looked at Lottie thoughtfully.

'I don't know,' she said. 'I can never make up my mind. She's happy here. She's used to us and she loves Sister and Bailey. Maybe it would be the same to her wherever she was so long as people were kind to her.'

'But how can she be happy?' I said. 'What about all the things she hears and sees going on around her in a ward like this?' I was thinking of the senility, the deaths, and the strange mumblings and mutterings that haunt every chronic ward during the night, and often during the daytime as well.

'Who's to tell,' said Brown. 'She probably doesn't even notice them. There's probably a merciful blind spot that people like her get which stops them from seeing the things they don't want to see, or even hearing the things they don't want to hear. Perhaps it's all part of some sort of plan to keep them happy.' She paused for a moment, then went on. There was a hint of defiance in her voice as if she was ashamed of saying such fanciful things. 'Well, there has to be something, doesn't there? If there wasn't, people couldn't bear half the things they have to bear, especially on a ward like this. How could Mrs Mackenzie possibly keep sane if she was aware of all the things that were happening to her?'

I thought about Mrs Mackenzie. She was an attractive, intelligent woman in her early sixties. Her devoted husband and family had visited her regularly since she had the stroke six years ago that had paralysed her from the waist down. When the sister and I were doing the things that had to be done for her that morning she had kept us amused with accounts of the funny things that had happened to her doctor son in his surgery the week before and the shocking things her daughter told her happened regularly in the school where she valiantly tried to instil knowledge into a class of unruly boys. Mrs Mackenzie had seemed quite undisturbed by the things that were being done for her below the waist, except for groaning a little every time we turned her from one side to the other. She certainly seemed to have the blind spot that Brown had talked about, which kept her from a full realization of her loss of control over bowels and bladder, and also kept her happy.

I had been astonished by the depth of feeling that Brown had put into her voice. As far as I could remember we had always been too busy in the past to stand around discussing any master plan there might be for keeping the patients happy. We left that sort of thing for visiting priests and parsons to ponder over while we got on with the poulticing and purging, the scouring of bedpans and the daily domestic duties, which were as much part of our work as attending to the patients' needs, and took up as much of our time. It suddenly seemed that the patients had become more important than the meticulous width of the turnback of the top sheet on their beds, or the weekly scrubbing of lockers and cupboards. I welcomed the change in attitude but found it hard to adjust to. There were many times during the next few weeks when I was to find myself wondering which was the more important: that a bed should be properly made and well tucked in, or that the patient lying in it should be comfortable. I had been trained by sisters who often resented time spent making the patients comfortable if there were bed springs waiting to be polished. I had already noticed that on this ward the bed springs were never polished. Neither were they given a daily dusting.

Bailey walked towards us down the ward looking very pleased with herself.

'Where on earth have you been?' asked Brown.

Bailey smiled happily.

'I've been telling Jennie about the film I went to see last night. She really enjoyed it. She laughed all the way through until it got to the sad bit at the end, then she cried. It was terribly sad when those two lovers walked hand in hand into the sunset before he got killed by the sheriff's men who mistook him for a baddie.'

She and Lynch exchanged a few words about the sad ending to an otherwise funny film, then we disbanded and Lottie went back to her sweeping while the rest of us got on with the afternoon work. Listening to Bailey had astonished me as much as listening to Brown. The most astonishing thing about it was that nobody seemed to doubt that making Jennie laugh or cry over a film was worth the time spent for the therapeutic benefits she derived from it. Bailey had taken her, however briefly, into a world that was as escapist for her as it had been for everybody else watching the film. The lovers she wept over were as real to her as the flowers she could see from her chair.

It took time for me to change my way of thinking. I fidgeted to get on with the next patient when Bailey, Brown and Lynch stood listening attentively to what the previous patient had to say. It was a topsy-turvy nursing world I had come back to, very different from the way it was when I was a full-time nurse.

The doctor arrived on the ward unheralded and unwelcomed, just as the Matron had arrived in the morning. He stuck his head round a set of screens behind which Bailey and I were prettying up a granny ready for him to go over her chest with a stethoscope. The granny was expressing great concern at having to have her nightdress removed and a clean one put on in front of an imaginary multitude of men who were gathered round her bed eagerly awaiting the strip show. The very young doctor who put his head round the screens was clearly not one of the multitude. Granny beamed at him, then tore off her nightdress with a shameless abandon that might have interested him more if she had been sixty years younger and lying in a bed somewhere outside his professional stamping ground. He coaxed her to lie down and keep quiet while he ran the stethoscope over her chest, then tickled her into girlish submission while he slipped the clean nightdress on to her thin old body. At the end of it all, the old lady sank back on her pillows with a sigh of satisfaction, implying that it had been a great deal nicer to have a handsome young man putting her into her nightdress than two interfering young women trying to take her out of it. The doctor wore a smug look on his face that told Bailey and me how much better he thought he was at doing our job than we were. He gave the granny a gentle farewell smile, then he and I proceeded to do the round.

For a while everything went smoothly. The doctor had none of the awesome majesty that I had learned to associate with doctors in the past. He showed no sign of wanting me to bow down and worship him, though I was quite ready to at the first indication that he expected it. He asked me whether I thought we ought to step up the strength of the tablets that Ella was on for her epilepsy, and confessed that Sally-who-was-nearly-a-hundred terrified him when she pounded her stick on the floor, as she did when he asked her to put out her tongue for him. He said he had no doubt at all that the moment his back was turned she would poke her tongue out at him anyway so why she couldn't do it so that he could see whether it was coated or not, he didn't know. Both of us agreed that it was probably because of the stubborn streak in her, which made her unwilling to do anything that anybody asked her to do.

The strange new familiarity between doctor and nurse that had taken the place of the chilly aloofness I was more accustomed to coping with confused and embarrassed me at first. I had always liked things to be the way I was used to them being. Any new departure threw me into a state of uncertainty. I would have been happier if he had stared down at me from his six foot two of superior medical knowledge and barked out his orders, instead of looking at me for suggestions when a patient told us she hadn't slept for a week when we knew from the night nurse's report that she regularly had to be wakened up to be given her sleeping tablets. But as the round progressed I grew in confidence. I gently nudged him into ordering an aperient for Agnes, who said she hadn't 'been' for days, and suggested that Ada, who was 'going' all the time should be put on something that would give her and us less frequent journeys down the corridor.

Then suddenly the confidence was shattered. The relationship that had slowly grown up between us took a temporary setback. We had reached bed number twenty from where the blood was to be taken when the ground started slipping away beneath my feet. I had laid up the tray paying strictest attention to detail and going over it many times to ensure that nothing would be found wanting when the doctor wanted it. There were syringes, needles, swabs and towels and everything else I could remember arranging on a tray for just such an occasion. I was just starting to congratulate myself on the speed at which I had got back into the swing of things when the doctor gave a grunt. At first I thought the grunt was his way of showing approval at my efforts, but when he gave another grunt I knew at once that translated it would have some deep significance, and the most likely significance was that I had left something vital off the tray. Instead of bringing my new-found confidence to the fore and asking for a translation of the grunt, I looked wildly round, then turned and raced up the ward to go in aimless search of whatever it had indicated was urgently required by the doctor.

I was still going madly through cupboards and drawers in the medical room when Brown walked in.

She gazed round at the scattered surgical appliances and rubber goods that littered the floor and at the bottles and boxes that were stacked on the trolleys.

'What on earth are you looking for?' she asked, even she losing a little of her usual calm at the sight.

'I don't know,' I said making a last desperate attempt at finding it.

'Then why are you looking for it?' she asked in reasonable tones.

I explained about the grunt and the confusion it had thrown me into and she stormed up the ward with me in tow. She drew up sharply at bed number twenty and fixed the doctor with a stern eye.

'The staff nurse didn't understand a word you were saying,' she said, 'and neither do I half the time. Why you doctors can't speak up instead of muttering to yourselves all the time I really don't know. It's getting to be as bad as your writing. It's a wonder more people aren't killed with being given the wrong things. What was it you were grunting for?'

The doctor shuffled uncomfortably, then apologized to me for the grunt and told Brown what it had been intended to mean. It was one of the new skin preparation things I had read about in the nursing journals but had never come across before. If I had scrabbled about in the medical room for a week I would never have associated the grunt with the name of the product.

Brown went off at a leisurely pace to get it for him and when she came back she told him in a forgiving sort of way that there would be a cup of coffee waiting for him in the office after he had finished the round – and for the staff nurse as well, she added kindly. I could only stand and wonder that anybody of a lower order than a sister should be brave enough to question a doctor's grunts and bold enough to promise him a cup of coffee when he had finished the round. We took the blood from bed number twenty without further grunts, and by the time it was labelled and ready to be dispatched to the path lab I had almost forgotten what had gone before.

It took a small incident at the ward door to throw me back into confusion. I had followed the doctor at a respectful distance while we finished the round, then followed him again at a respectful distance while we walked down the ward to the wash basin. I had hovered over him holding the towel for him to dry his hands on, then I stood at an even more respectful distance waiting for him to precede me through the ward door. His polite insistence that I should go through it first and my determination that I should follow him resulted in us getting tightly jammed in the doorway together. We were a long time extricating ourselves from a difficult situation.

The coffee that Brown had promised us was waiting

for us on the office table, but I was too unnerved to drink it. Lottie, who had sidled into the office behind us, drank mine for me while she was having a cosy little chat with the doctor about the twinges that had been troubling her lately. When she went away with the empty cups she seemed quite satisfied with his grunted diagnosis of the twinge. I envied her the ease that allowed her to drink coffee, chat to a doctor, drop hairpins around and waggle a cigarette in her mouth all at the same time. It was an ease that I could never enjoy.

When I told Brown about the tussle I'd had with the doctor at the ward door, she laughed at the picture it conjured up.

'But we don't do things like that these days,' she told me, after she had stopped laughing. 'It's only the most senior consultants who expect to be treated like gods, and even they have started to climb down a bit lately. Most of them stand back to let us go through a door first, and those that don't have to be taken down a peg or two before they get too big for their boots.'

I couldn't see myself taking down any pegs. I had been trailing behind doctors for too long to suddenly start charging in front of them. I knew my place. I had been trained to know it by a succession of sisters who were sticklers for ward etiquette. I had the greatest difficulty for a long time forcing myself not to address the most junior houseman as 'sir'.

At half-past three I started plucking up courage to tell the others that I was going off duty. I was guiltily aware that I was going at a time when they needed me most. Though the grannies had been brought in off the verandah, they were still sitting in their chairs waiting to be put back to bed. Putting them back and doing all the other things that had to be done before the suppers came up to the ward would keep Bailey, Lynch and Brown fully occupied, and they would be kept just as busy after the suppers were given out until the time they went off duty. The thought that I would be idling my time away at home while they were working their fingers to the bone kept me hanging about when I should have been over at the locker room putting my outdoor things on.

None of them seemed to be as worried about my impending departure as I was. Lynch said she'd see me in the morning if her mother managed to get over in time to let her do the early shift. Bailey said it was her day off tomorrow, thank the Lord, so she wouldn't be seeing me until Wednesday, and Brown told me not to worry about going off duty just when the worst of the evening work was starting. They were quite used to it, she said. All it would mean was that the full-timers and the late-shift workers would die of heart attacks and strokes through having to work doubly hard because I wasn't there. For a moment I thought she meant it and my heart sank, then I saw she was only joking and I said 'Cheerio' to them and went. But, as I walked across to the locker room, I couldn't help worrying a little and thinking that having to run a hospital with so many nurses whose first priorities were their homes and families must be giving an awful lot of people an awful lot of headaches. I hoped the patients weren't getting too big a share of them.

The locker room was buzzing with part-timers. They were tearing off their uniform coats and throwing on their raincoats with a feverish haste which told me that they, like me, had urgent things waiting for them when they got home. Some were having a quick draw at a cigarette and changing their shoes at the same time, others were checking shopping lists for things they had to buy on their way home. Those who passed me on their way out as I was going in gave me a curious stare but hurried on, too pushed for time to have any to spare for me. The two who were flinging things about in the lockers on either side of mine muttered a greeting but went on flinging things about. There was too much for part-timers to think about at half-past three than exchanging polite chat with each other. I changed my shoes, tore off my uniform coat, put on my outdoor things and left the locker room. It seemed a long time since I had walked into it that morning.

All I wanted to do when I eventually got home was to throw my aching body down on one chair and put my tortured feet up on another. But I knew that such self-indulgent lotus eating was not for me: I was a wife and a mother, not a full-time nurse with nothing to do when she came off duty but put her feet up. I rushed round to Selina's, thanked her for having the children and dragged them away from the television set.

The children were very annoyed at having to be dragged away just as things had started hotting up for Andy Pandy and his little blonde siren, Looby Loo, who played innocent games with him which invariably ended in poor old pyjama-clad Andy having to climb into his box bed alone. When they had stopped sulking over this untimely end to their entertainment, I listened lovingly while they gave me a detailed account of the terrible things that had happened to them at school that day. I cooked the dinner, collected the eggs, welcomed my husband home from work and listened lovingly while he gave me a detailed account of all the terrible things that had happened to him at the office that day. Then I washed up the dinner things, bathed the children, put them to bed and heard their prayers, and threatened them with the terrible things that would happen to them if they so much as stirred after I had kissed them and said good night for the sixth time. I did a bit of surface cleaning, washed a couple of pairs of socks through ready for the morning, and finally gave the breadwinner his supper, which he ate wearily before he stumbled upstairs to bed.

It was only after I had shot the last bolt and turned out the last light that it occurred to me that nobody had asked me what sort of day I had had. If any of them remembered that it was my first day back at work, nobody had thought it worthy of a mention. I felt a small stab of resentment at their lack of interest in my third role, but I was asleep before the stab had time to grow into a bleeding wound. I had had a very busy day – and there was another busy day waiting for me tomorrow.

Chapter Seven

IF, AS ANYBODY who is even remotely connected with the theatre maintains, the smell of greasepaint stays forever in the blood (or, more aptly, lodges permanently somewhere up the nose), then the smell that pervades a hospital ward must slowly but surely seep into the circulatory system of a nurse. Even the sluice has an emanation that lingers in the memory long after it is banished from the atmosphere by an air freshener. The pungent odour of disinfectants and the more earthy scent of other things earns the sluice a place of its own in hospital nostalgia: more lasting than the smell of the nurses' home, where along every corridor stalk the ghosts of a million meals of cabbage stew and boiled suet puddings; more abiding than the smell of the laundry which, in spite of the newly installed modern machinery, still has traces of the steamy soapy days when the laundry maids boiled the hospital linen as devotedly as the cooks boiled the suet puddings.

The day after I started back to work I suddenly found myself at home with smells, even enjoying them in a special sort of way. They had been part of my life for so long that getting back to them again gave me a feeling of deep content. The content was to stay with me, making the years that I spent as a part-time nurse some of the happiest and most rewarding of any I had spent in hospital.

The family took longer to get used to them. Their content ranged from the mildly curious to the frankly critical.

'Pooh,' said the children, stepping closer to get the full impact of the essence of hospital that I brought home with me. 'You do smell funny since you started going to work. You smell like a lot of medicine and things.' The 'things' were things they could never properly identify.

Their father wasn't quite so diplomatic. 'Phew,' he would say, stepping back and holding his nose. 'You do smell awful. You've reeked of disinfectant and things ever since you went back to work.' He sometimes put a name to the 'things'. The names were usually rude and had to be used in front of the children in lowered tones, or not used at all until they had gone to bed. We were still living in an age when rude words, like the facts of life, were picked up by children in school playgrounds and rarely, if ever, in their own homes.

Their father could have been right about the names he put to the things. Whatever is done to eliminate the smells from a sluice, they can linger on the person as well as in the memory, clinging closely and, like all clinging things, more noticeable to those at the receiving end than to those who give them off.

But soon the family were accepting them as they were having to accept all the other small inconveniences they suffered by having a part-time nurse instead of a full-time wife and mother. Buttons were put into button holes, though not always into the right ones; shoelaces were tied and even the occasional cup of tea got poured out with a minimum of guidance from me. I showed the youngest how to hold a duster in her tiny hand and run it up and down chair legs and across the top of the sideboard. I stood the eldest on a stool, high enough to enable her to see into the sink while she was doing the washing up for me. I also taught them both a little rhyme to repeat when they were making their beds: 'First the foot and then the head, that's the way to make a bed,' they chanted, while they did hospital corners with the counterpane and turned down the top sheet to a prescribed width. Cooperation and organization became key words, of vital importance to the smooth running of the household.

I had spent a long time after I passed my Finals learning how to delegate responsibility, and learning that delegating responsibility meant pushing the jobs one least liked doing on to those who had no option but to get on and do them without too much audible complaint. I was a great deal better at it now than I was then. The children were younger than the probationers, and I was their mother: I had the whip hand. Though I seldom raised it, their fear that I would if driven kept the complaints inaudible, at least to my ears. But however tactfully I coaxed and however much I bullied, I could never tempt Daddy with a duster. He stood on the sidelines watching the three women in his life delegating and cooperating madly while he waited more or less patiently until it was his turn to get a little of their attention. Women's Lib wasn't around when I needed it. Only the helpless, clinging little women were truly liberated, and theirs was a different kind of liberation from that which their daughters were to picket for later if they were the picketing militant types. Their velvety hands were encased in mitts of steel. They never had to climb on chairs to reach for something off a top shelf, or do any of the nasty dirty jobs they didn't like doing. They had hubbies who rushed forward at the smallest cry to get the jam off the top shelf or to bring in a scuttle of coal. But in an average household like ours the fact that the man was the breadwinner gave him the undisputed right to doze in a chair while his number one woman swept the floor around him, making sure that he was never disturbed by the sweeping brush. That his number one woman also went out to work was never a valid excuse for there being no clean socks in the clean sock drawer when they were called for. The busy day she had so blithely skipped through could never compete in the sympathy stakes with the busy day that had almost given him an ulcer.

While my loved ones were adjusting to me going out to work, I was having almost as much trouble making my own adjustments. The changing attitudes that had troubled me so much on my first day back continued to trouble me for a long time. When I was stopped in my tracks while I was careering up the ward one day and reminded by a patient that I was now a public servant, paid out of public funds exactly like a postman, I had to ask Brown what the patient was talking about. I asked not because I minded being coupled with a postman, but because the patient had implied that he and I were a burden on the State and I had no wish to be a burden on anybody, and certainly not on the State.

'It's the new National Health Service,' Brown explained.

'But what's that got to do with me and the postman?' I asked her. She didn't answer for a moment. She was struggling with a backrest that collapsed every time she got the patient in the bed comfortably resting against it. I stopped asking questions and tightened the screws of the backrest while she propped up the patient. It was a curious thing about Brown that if there were two jobs to be done and she and I were doing them, she usually ended up with the job that more directly involved the patient while I was left to tighten screws, turn on taps or shift apparatus about. I had noticed this when we worked together on nights at the Sanatorium, but it was done in a natural way, with no intention of wounding my pride, so my pride was never wounded.

When the backrest screws were secure enough to support the patient, we rearranged pillows and straightened the draw sheet and then Brown told me about the Health Service and the changes it had made in the patients' attitudes to nurses and doctors.

'Before it started, most of the patients, especially those in the Municipal hospitals, thought that nurses were a bit special even if we weren't. But now that they think they pay our wages out of their insurance stamp, they feel they have a right to criticize us and demand value for their money. Instead of regarding us as Florence Nightingales and angels of mercy, they know we are ordinary people like them and get paid for what we do instead of working for love. They feel just the same about the National Health doctors.' She didn't sound too upset at the changing attitudes that were creeping into the system. She was a very fair-minded woman and even I had to admit that getting paid two shillings and twopence an hour as a staff nurse, part-time and non-resident, must be putting an enormous strain on the nation's resources.

I knew that what she told me was right. I had read articles in the papers, and letters to the Editor, criticizing the newly structured Health Service. Some of the letters, signed 'Irate Patient', had gone so far as to demand that nurses should be made to stop clanking bedpans in the night when the patients were trying to sleep. For as long as I could remember, and for a long time before that, nurses had been clanking bedpans in the night when the patients were trying to sleep, but nobody had thought of writing a letter to the Editor about it before.

I had even read somewhere about a family that was threatening to sue a doctor for allowing one of their relatives to die when he should have been keeping him alive. I couldn't be as detached about such things as Brown appeared to be. I had been trained to think of a doctor as being as irreproachable as he was unap-proachable. That anyone should question what he did, and especially in the newspapers, could only undermine the faith his patients needed to have in the man who strived, however unsuccessfully, to keep them alive. If he occasionally failed to keep them alive that was a risk that everybody had to take. He was only human after all, despite the fund of specialized knowledge he had managed to pick up on his way through medical school.

The new National Health Service was affecting the nurses' attitude to nursing as much as it affected the patients' attitude to those who were caring for them. Probationer nurses were not called probationers any more. They were now 'students'. The name gave the juniors status they didn't have when they were brow-beaten little probationers holed up in a sluice for most of their early training. Being students entitled them to have their lectures under a block system and in the hospital time instead of during their off duty, or in the middle of the day when they were on nights. Getting up in the middle of the day to sit in a lecture room yawning over a collection of dry bones or listening to a dreary talk on duodenal ulcers had never been a favourite pursuit with probationers. They missed most of the lectures by not being able to keep their eyes open while the sister tutor was talking. It was some-times a serious drawback to them when they sat for their exams.

'You have nobody but yourselves to blame,' said Brown acidly, when I mentioned some of these things to her. 'You should have stood up for yourselves a bit more instead of lying down under it and letting every-body walk over you.'

I had never thought of our obedience to the rules as being walked over. I had thought of it as respecting our seniors and keeping on the right side of the sister so that she wouldn't be too scathing about us in her ward report. But Brown didn't see it that way. When she told me that some of the students had actually climbed on to a coal cart in Trafalgar Square and waved banners about demanding a minimum wage of five pounds a week I refused to believe it. I knew my mother wouldn't have believed it either. She was as firm in her belief that nurses were ladies as my father was in his belief that the earth was flat. She would most certainly never have sent me off to be a nurse if she had thought there was any risk of me ending up in a coal cart in Trafalgar Square waving banners about. I would have had to be a teacher instead.

'Some of the students even belong to a trade union now,' said Brown, shocking me into further disbelief. Trade unions were for men. They were the mainstay of strikes, industrial disputes and other means of bringing the country to a standstill. Who, I asked myself, would dream of leaving patients to fend for themselves while they rushed away to have a strike? The idea was unthinkable.

But in spite of the feelings I had against the student nurses who were at last standing up for their own rights and mine as well, I had no qualms about accepting the extra money we all got, partly because of the stand they took. Though my conscience told me that I should refuse the award on the grounds that I disapproved of the way it was won, I had no trouble in persuading my conscience that it was the Whitley Council that had won it for us – and so it might have been, but not without a push in the back from the students. The Lady with the Lamp might have winced at the coal cart but she would surely have admired the courage that got it into Trafalgar Square. Even Nelson must have looked down at it with a compassionate eye.

However much I worried about the changing attitudes that I was coming up against all the time, I worried even more over the changing techniques that I was having to get myself acquainted with. For a week or two after I went back to work I lay awake at night haunted by the fear that the penicillin I had given the day before might not have been penicillin at all but something entirely different, and maybe something that did more harm than good. One glass phial in the medical room looked very much the same as all the other glass phials that were brought to the ward in batches by the dispensary porters. Mistaking one for another could only be avoided by careful scrutiny of the small print. I tended to spend so much time scrutinizing the small print that the next injection was almost due before I had given the first.

When I had finally managed to persuade myself that, with all the checking and rechecking I had done on the penicillin, it couldn't possibly have been anything else,

I stopped worrying about it, plumped up my pillows, turned over – and promptly started worrying about the sterile water I'd used for diluting the penicillin. Could I have concocted a lethal mixture instead of the magical antibiotic that Alexander Fleming had started dreaming up as long ago as 1928? Would the patients I had given the injection to still be there when I went on duty in the morning or would their beds be empty or filled with a fresh lot of patients, and a posse of police be awaiting me, handcuffs at the ready?

That none of the nightmares came true was almost entirely due to my fear that they might. I could get within striking distance of a patient's bottom, syringe poised, then break out into a cold sweat of panic, pull the sheets up over the bared bottom and rush back to the medical room for another quick check on the discarded phials. Giving an injection of one of the new antibiotics was almost as frightening for me when I first went back to work as giving an injection of a dangerous drug had been when I was doing my training. In those days it had required mathematical genius to work out the correct dosage of morphia, heroin and other such deadly substances. I was never much good at maths.

Not all the different techniques I had to learn kept me awake at night. Some merely astonished me; others mortified me. The mortifying ones were those that I was expected to know about and didn't. When somebody handed me a stethoscope and walked away, leaving me to take a patient's blood pressure, I looked at the stethoscope and at the rest of the apparatus and hadn't the courage to confess that I had never taken anybody's blood pressure before. I had learned the hows, the whys and the wherefores in the lecture room, but in the final analysis it had always been a doctor who pumped up the bag and recorded the reading. It was the nurse's role to reassure the patient and loosen the armband before the circulation stopped and the arm fell off.

'You wrap it round me arm, then listen to me heart,' said the patient helpfully, rolling up her sleeve ready for the great adventure. I knew that it wasn't quite as simple as that, but I plugged the stethoscope into my ears and pumped. I was greatly relieved when Brown noticed the dilemma I was in and came across to rescue me from it. She did it so tactfully that nobody would ever have suspected that I hadn't actually taken a blood pressure before. Even the patient was fooled, for which I was doubly grateful. It would never have done to let her run away with the idea that a nurse wearing a navy blue belt and navy blue epaulettes had to be shown how to do such a simple thing by an assistant nurse.

Brown made it her business, while she was showing me, to see that the next time someone handed me a stethoscope I would know exactly what to do with it.

Because it was Brown who showed me I felt less embarrassed at having to be shown. I would have died with shame if it had been Bailey. Student nurses were whipping round the ward taking blood pressures with as much confidence as probationer nurses had once whipped round the wards removing the nits from the patients' heads. That, and cleaning their teeth, had been absorbing occupations when we weren't scouring enamel bedpans or washing down walls. Bailey hadn't scoured a bedpan since the day she became a nurse. The bedpans were popped into a machine, levers were pushed and pulled, and hey presto the bedpan came out clean. It was an age of miracles we were living in. Bailey hadn't washed a ward wall down either; there were people employed to do that, and it was no longer thought to be an essential part of a nurse's training. Bailey knew more about nursing in her eighteen months as a student than I had known after three years. But I could have taught her a thing or two about buffing a floor or scraping a spittoon. They were the things we were more accomplished in than taking blood pressures. They were the things the sisters had insisted were done properly.

It was Brown who rescued me again when the patient in bed number twenty, where I had suffered my first humiliation, had to have a blood transfusion. As I had feared on my first day back at work, because I was State Registered everybody expected me to know everything. Setting up a blood transfusion was one of the things that should have come easy to me. It didn't. I still remembered the mess I made of it when an examiner asked me to set up for one on the day that I sat my Finals. Many of the things I put on the trolley were never needed, and many that were indispensable I had cheerfully dispensed with. The wonder was that I ever passed the exam. I must have known something about something to offset the little I knew about setting up for a blood transfusion.

After I had sunk my pride enough to confess to Brown that with the passage of time I had become a little rusty on blood transfusions, she took me down to the medical room and showed me several small packages that were stacked on the shelves. I had noticed them there before and wondered what they were.

'It's different now,' she said, waving a hand at the packages. 'They send most of it up from the dispensary already sterilized and assembled.' And indeed they did. It was all in packages, wrapped like an instant dinner, needing only to be unwrapped when the doctor asked for them. It had been simplified and made so foolproof that even I couldn't go wrong, nor ever did I. I would have given the examiner far fewer headaches if the system had been in operation when I sat my Finals.

But in spite of having to admit that a nurse's lot had been made easier in a number of ways over the years, I still had certain reservations about some things. It was almost twenty years since I had done my training, and I was as much of an old-timer as I was a part-timer. I had been taught to cosset pneumonia with poultices and to bring abscesses to a painful head with fomentations. Now there was a magic wand being waved over everything which had made the poultices and fomentations as old-fashioned as leeches and cupping. The wand was called antibiotics. It was waved so often and for so many things that it seemed in danger of losing its magic powers. When a wave of flu struck the ward we spent our days sawing the tops off glass phials and running up and down with syringes.

'We never seem to do any proper nursing,' I grumbled to Brown one morning when we were in the medical room boiling up a fresh lot of syringes for the next lot of injections, and searching for hypodermic needles with no fish hooks on the end; disposable needles and syringes still had to make their debut. When they did the patients suffered a lot less anguish from having their bottoms pierced with blunt needles or with needles that turned up at the end enough to make a jagged hole in the most leathery skin.

'What are you talking about?' asked Brown, throwing another load of enamel ware into the sterilizer and slamming down the lid.

'Well, at least we used to nurse people when there weren't any antibiotics,' I said, running the piston up and down the barrel of a syringe a few times to loosen it.

'All we seem to do these days is stick needles in people. I sometimes feel more like a technician than a nurse.'

'I don't agree with you,' she said, wiping steam off her spectacles. 'It's still nursing. We do it in a different way, that's all, and a lot better way, in my opinion. Think of the women on the gynae wards who used to die of septicaemia and puerperal fever, and the breast abscesses and the pneumonias, and the weeks it took to clear up a little thing like an ear infection and the simple things that children used to die of.'

I thought of them while I was rolling a few fresh swabs ready for filling a drum.

'But we give antibiotics for everything,' I said, tearing at the roll of cotton wool. 'What happens when everybody's used to them and they stop working? People will start dying again then.'

'I don't think we need worry about that,' said Brown. 'Somebody's bound to think up a fresh lot when these stop working. We're hardly likely to go back to linseed poultices and vinegar and brown paper.'

'No, I suppose you're right,' I said, putting a fresh pile of dressing towels on to the trolley.

As the months went by I gained in confidence. I was able to give things without having to check so often on the things I was giving. I managed to muster enough courage to walk through a door in front of a doctor, and I had even been known to ask for a repeat of his grunt when I hadn't understood the first time. But there were still moments when I wished Selina had never suggested that I got myself a job and went out to work. One of these moments came when I was at a low ebb and not in full control of the situation. This time Brown was no help at all. It was she who was partly responsible for creating the situation.

Chapter Eight

THE REMARKABLE ABILITY I had to turn a blind eye to all but the most glaring deficiencies in the housework had been a great help to me since I went back to work. Although I sometimes felt guilty when I heard other part-timers tell of the struggle they had to keep the floors at home clean enough to eat off, my floors never reached that standard. They fell so far below it that a slice of toast landing buttered side down usually came up only fit to be thrown to the birds. When I lightly brushed aside the fluff by asking the family which of them would want to eat off the floors anyway, at least one of them hinted that, though he might never want to, the thought that he could if he ever got the urge held certain attractions for him. The criticism implied in the hint threw me into a frenzy of activity aimed at proving that such perfection was well within my scope. When the frenzy had burnt itself out we reverted to a more normal state of dusty disorder.

As well as the advantage of the blind eye, I had another ally in the shape of a large tapestry bag I had been bullied into buying by a high-powered saleswoman at a Christmas bazaar. She called it a reticule; we christened it 'the bag'. It was kept in a little cubbyhole in the kitchen, and into it went the bits and pieces and odds and ends which if left lying about long enough became a serious threat to peaceful co-existence. It grew fat on a daily diet of odd socks, one or two items in need of repair and a number of other things too intimate to mention. The bag became the family friend. Brown used it one morning to make the small dent in my growing confidence.

The day of my discomfiture had got off to a bad start. Nothing went right from the moment the alarm clock woke us up. The children had one of their memory lapses which sent them helter-skeltering upstairs and downstairs searching for that which they could not find. It took a couple of sharp slaps on their chubby little legs and a few harsh words to restore their memory and lead them to whatever it was they were looking for. As is usual in such trying times, the things they sought were in the place they should have been looked for from the beginning.

Neither of the adult members of the family was in any mood for compromise, and even the budgerigar stood first on one leg and then on the other, tucking his head under his wing until the storm abated. Joey was no fool. His little bird brain told him that, however much he tweeted to be told what a pretty boy he was, there wasn't a hope of anybody stopping at the cage to

140

scratch his downy little head and pander to his ego, so he wisely kept his beak shut, which was more than anybody else did in the house that morning.

I had managed to survive the war, and even emerged from it the victor, and was just stepping out of the battlefield to go to work, when I remembered that the cupboard was almost bare and that things would have to be bought on my way home that afternoon if the family were to eat at suppertime. I turned back into the chaos of the kitchen and looked for a small bag, big enough to hold a pound of sausages or a tin of something that could be turned into a quick meal if I came home too tired to experiment with *haute cuisine*. There was no small bag. The only bag I could lay my hands on in the limited time available to me was the reticule, the faithful family friend, the receptacle for our droppings which, without it, would have been left to litter the floor or take up valuable space on all the working tops. It was already a little bloated with the morning's contributions, but I added a pen, a pencil and a pair of scissors to the small collection and went to work, going at the double, to make up for time lost.

The ward was in a turmoil. The doorway was blocked with two ambulance men separated by a stretcher. From the snatches of conversation I picked up while I waited to gain access, I gathered that the patient on the stretcher had decided that she didn't want to come into hospital after all, thank you very much; she just wanted the two kind gentlemen to take her back home where she belonged. I pushed my way through the little group that was talking out the problem and went to report to the ward sister. She had a wild look in her eyes. Lottie stood before her arguing furiously about something, scattering hairpins everywhere and waving her sweeping brush about in a most endangering way.

At the far end of the ward a full set of screens arranged round a bed told me that Mrs Green had died, either in the night or early that morning. I was neither surprised nor even sorry that she had died. Mrs Green had been waiting to die since the day they told her that her husband would no longer be coming to see her from the men's ward where he was taken after the outside authorities decided that he and Mrs Green were no longer able to take care of each other and would be better in hospital. Lottie had different ideas.

'They might just as well have left them at home,' she said, when we heard that the old man had died only a week or two after they were admitted. 'They'd looked after each other all those years, another week or two wouldn't have made much difference, and they would have been happier together instead of having to be brought here and put into separate wards. The district nurse could have gone in to see how they were getting on.'

We pointed out to Lottie that it was the authorities' choice, and they knew best what was good for old people, but she still argued. She hadn't much respect for authority. She flouted it whenever it got in the way of her doing the things she wanted to do.

Halfway down the ward, Bailey and Lynch were almost giving themselves hernias trying to get Mrs Small up, and on the other side was a less enclosing set of screens behind which somebody had to be doing something that required privacy. I hoped it was a patient on a bedpan and not a doctor dealing with drama. Glancing round at the scene I guessed it was going to be one of those days when I would wonder why I had stopped being just a housewife, with nothing to do, and taking from morning to night to do it. Then I thought of the bills, and the pay packet I got at the end of the week which went a long way towards paying them. I threw back my shoulders and became part of the turmoil.

'Thank heavens you're here,' said the sister, making me suddenly glad that I was. 'It's a bit hectic at the moment with one thing and another. There's the new patient to be warded when the ambulance men have finished sorting her out, the mortuary porter will be here any minute to take Mrs Green away and the doctor is getting Mrs Love ready to have a test meal. I think you'd better go and relieve Brown. She's with the doctor. Tell her to give Bailey and Lynch a hand with Mrs Small. That woman gets fatter every day.'

She hurried off to give the ambulance men her support, and I walked up the ward throwing a look of sympathy at Bailey and Lynch as I passed them. They needed all the sympathy they could get, but they would have appreciated another pair of strong arms more than they appreciated the sympathy.

Mrs Small was extremely large. Despite the thousand-calorie diet she was supposed to be on she still managed to gain a steady two pounds a week. Rumour had it that Lottie was responsible for Mrs Small's failure to respond to the diet and shrink away until she was nothing but a bag of bones. Lottie was very fond of Mrs Small. She said she thought it was a crying shame that a nice old lady like her should have to sit nibbling a lettuce leaf while everybody else was tucking into lovely stew with globules of grease floating on the top and indifferently cooked rice pudding. Though she was never caught red-handed, Lottie was the prime suspect of bringing in the packet of biscuits and slabs of chocolate that Mrs Small foraged for in the middle of the night, and even during the day when she thought nobody was looking. As fast as we cleared out the thousands of extra calories, more found their way into her locker, and the fatter Mrs Small got.

Getting her up in the morning was a miracle of team

work; putting her into the bath called for muscular strength that Charles Atlas would have been proud of. His boast that by following his methods of body-building the follower would develop legs like tree trunks and mighty biceps paled almost to insignificance beside the walking advertisement for body-building that anybody could become after weeks of grappling with Mrs Small. Bailey and Lynch were having to dig their heels in deeply to get a grip on the mountain of quivering flesh.

Brown seemed as pleased to see me as the sister had been. With standing in one place behind the screens with the doctor for so long, her arches were beginning to fall a little. Brown's arches were by no means her strongest feature. Considering how often they let her down it said a great deal for her determination to be a nurse that she had even got over the first few weeks of working in a hospital. She was standing first on one leg and then on the other, just as the budgerigar had done at home.

'Thank God you've come,' she whispered hoarsely behind the doctor's back. She nodded towards him and the patient he was leaning over. 'He's getting ready for a test meal.'

'I know,' I whispered back. 'The sister told me. Why is he having to do it and not one of us?' Trying to coax a patient to swallow a length of rubber tubing in preparation for a test meal was a task that was usually assigned to a nurse who had learned all about

'Fractional Test Meals' in the lecture room and was good at persuading patients to swallow twenty inches of rubber tubing. There had to be some very good reason for a doctor to demean himself by edging the tube inch by inch down the patient's throat.

'He had to do it,' said Brown, still whispering but getting more hoarse. 'She wouldn't let any of us near her, not even the sister. She threatened to bite us if we tried to put the tube in her mouth.'

The old lady had my sympathy. There were one or two things that I had seen done or learned to do while I was a nurse which would have troubled me a lot if they ever had to be done to me. But whether I would have gone so far as to bite the hand that was feeding me with the rubber tube was as debatable as whether the old lady could have managed it without her dentures in. They were soaking in Steradent on the locker waiting to be popped back into her mouth when the test meal was over. Without them her bite was to be feared considerably less than her bark.

The doctor straightened his back and turned to us. 'There aren't any scissors on the tray,' he said, sounding faintly irritable after the bad time the old lady had given him. Brown patted her pockets and looked at me. I patted my pockets and looked apologetically at the doctor. He was standing expectantly, gripping the visible end of the rubber tubing that the patient had at last been coaxed to swallow between the thumb and finger of one hand and a reel of adhesive tape in the other. A suitable length of tape needed to be cut, to attach the end of the tube to the patient's cheek. Unless it was stuck firmly into place there was a grave danger of the visible end disappearing suddenly into the patient's mouth or the invisible end popping up out of her stomach. Either disaster would mean that the whole thing must be gone through again. Whoever had laid the tray without a pair of scissors on it would have a lot to answer for if disaster happened.

'There's a pair of scissors in my bag in the ward cloakroom,' I hissed at Brown, glaring angrily at her for daring not to have a pair of scissors in her pocket when the doctor needed them. She glared at me for glaring at her, then went off to find the scissors while I stood beside the bed trying to avoid the doctor's eye. I had delegated the responsibility of finding the scissors to Brown and for once she hadn't wasted time arguing – which should have been a warning to me.

Within seconds she was back, not with the scissors but with the bag, the reticule, the faithful family friend. 'I couldn't find any scissors in it,' she said, and with a swift movement she tipped the bag upside down on the floor, depositing its contents at our feet. There was a curiously still moment while the three of us stared down at the heap. Bits and pieces jostled with odds and ends, unmatching

147

socks lay side by side with small items awaiting repair, and things too intimate to mention brought a blush to my cheeks. The skeleton that should have been in our cubbyhole at home had emerged to shame me. It was rattling its bones at our feet on the ward floor.

I stood covered with confusion for a moment. Then, bravely throwing off the confusion, I scooped up the scissors that had isolated themselves from the rest of the pile and handed them to the doctor. He tore his eyes from the unmentionables and cut off the strip of adhesive tape, while Brown, wearing the look of one who has avenged herself, kindly replaced the contents of the bag. Life went on almost as if the catastrophe had never occurred.

As with most catastrophes, the rumours about it spread and were greatly exaggerated. Though Brown might not have argued about being delegated the responsibility of finding the scissors she made me pay for it in other ways. She repeated the story until the odd socks were hyperbolized into a complete wardrobe of clothes, and the things too intimate to mention became things far more personal than would ever have found their way into our respectable tapestry reticule.

The jokes were just starting to wear a bit thin when other catastrophes happened to take our minds off trivialities and give us things to grieve over. But even then there were still a few things to laugh about.

Chapter Nine

THE YEAR HAD been full of incident. No sooner was January over and we were into February than the nation was thrown into confusion as sudden as it was shocking and sad. Things perked up a bit for a while, then we were thrown back into a different sort of confusion altogether.

The day they told us that the King had died peacefully in his sleep, even the very young were shaken by the news. In the stories and rhymes they spelt out letter by letter for themselves, or had read to them by somebody else it was only the bad kings that died. The good kings lived for ever, permanently royal, sitting on a golden throne and wearing a golden crown, with only a few short breaks while they rushed away to their counting houses or to eat tea in the parlour with the queen. It was difficult for the children to understand that the King who had died in the night was a good king and not so very different from ordinary men when he wasn't wearing his crown, though he had been doomed to die sooner than most ordinary men, except for those who had gone to the war and not come back.

The not-so-young were even more shaken by the news. They refused to believe at first that anything so awful should have been allowed to happen, especially at a time when so many magic wands were being waved to prevent such things happening. If a king could die of something as terrible as it was rumoured he had died of, then what hope was there of less high and mighty sufferers surviving it? If the most eminent doctors in the realm were powerless against disease, what chance was there of the overworked National Health doctors improving on their performance?

The King's death would have been easier for his subjects to accept if he had passed away in venerable old age instead of being struck down by a scourge that was almost as hush-hush in his own country as leprosy was in others. However obvious it might be to the neighbours that the man in the street was dying of cancer none of the neighbours would have been tactless enough to name the thing he was dying of when they were talking to the man's loved ones. They used evasive words and called it 'it'. And now rumour had it that the King had died of 'it'. The nation was stricken by disbelief as well as sorrow.

Those of us who were kindly invited into somebody's sitting room to watch the funeral on their television set were so affected by the grief of the King's widow and his two daughters that we refused the biscuit we were offered and let the tea get cold and missed much of the pageantry that marched side by side with the grief. Our eyes were so blurred with tears that we could hardly see the flickering greyish picture. The darkly veiled faces of our royal ladies were brought so far into the sitting room by the all-seeing hidden cameras that we might almost have been in Windsor ourselves. We were part of the action. Television was truly a remarkable invention.

But in the best tradition of 'The King is dead, long live the King', we soon stopped thinking of the poor dead King and started thinking of his eldest daughter instead. We cheered our new young Queen whenever she appeared in public, forgetting as we cheered that the reason she was the Queen was because her father had died, and, being so young, she must still be missing him. She had had to learn early her duty as a Queen. She knew she had to smile whether she felt like smiling or not just as she had to keep her shoes on in public however much her feet ached. I wasn't a queen, but I could have told her how much that would hurt. The comfortable pair of shoes I bought out of my first pay packet were never as comfortable as the shop girl who talked me into buying them had promised they would be. Corns that had sprouted on my first day back at work took root in my little toes to become infallible warnings of bad weather ahead.

We had just started to get used to singing 'God Save our Gracious Queen', instead of 'God Save our Gracious King' while we were scrambling out of our seats in the cinema in time to catch the last bus home, when we were again invited into somebody's sitting room for tea and biscuits. This time we drank the tea and dunked the biscuits while we watched the sadness of the faces of those whose sitting rooms had been washed away in the night by the torrent of water that roared over them. The rich amongst us who had not only got a television set but had been to Devon for holidays dwelt sadly on happy times spent at beauty spots that were now reduced to watery devastation. They brought out snapshots to show us what it had all been like before the rains came.

When the collecting boxes were brought round to swell the Flood Relief Fund even the poorest among us threw in as many sixpences and threepenny bits as we could afford, thankful to have got off so lightly with our own small flood. We also donated a few items of clothing that we had deluded ourselves into thinking had shrunk until our friendly enemies shattered the delusion by suggesting that the reason they were too tight for us was because we had put on so much weight lately.

But it was to be our turn next. Not for more floods, but for a thick impenetrable fog that hung over London and its outskirts, killing not far short of 5000 people before it went away, satisfied that it had done its worst.

The fog descended upon us while we were putting the final touches to the Christmas preparations. Though the war had been over for more than six years, the preparations were still something of a headache. There were queues for a lot of things, and long waits in the sweetshops while coupons were being cut out of ration books. The coupons entitled every man, woman and child in the country to rot their teeth, if they had any teeth, with five ounces of sweets each week. Even those who never ate sweets bought them: they were on the ration and it was a waste not to buy the things one was entitled to.

The prudent accumulated their coupons for Christmas. They fobbed their children off with promises of chocolate-filled stockings when they begged for a pre-Christmas jelly baby. The prudent also spent hours searching through wartime cook books and women's magazines looking for hints on how to make a little luxury go a long way. Given the proper processing a small tin of salmon could be stretched far enough to provide a feast for the family and still leave enough to fill sandwiches for supper. The few small Biblical fish that miraculously fed the 5000 with the help of a bit of bread would have fed more than 5000 if the cookery experts of the women's magazines had been around to offer help with the miracle. Not that the little fishes would have tasted anything like fish at the end of the processing, any more than the salmon tasted like salmon by the time it got into the sandwiches.

Even the not-so-prudent, of whom I was one, developed skills that were unique to the times. We had been developing them almost since the war began. We made sugar icings with so little sugar in them that the icing dripped steadily down the sides of the sunken cakes, leaving nothing to disguise the burnt top. We made tasteless marzipan with tasteless semolina and mock creams that were a mockery of anything that had ever come out of a dairy. The preparations we made for Christmas were made doubly exciting by the uncertainty of what they would look like when they were finished – or indeed what they would taste of if they tasted of anything.

There were other problems to give us headaches. The drapery stores ran out of the last-for-ever nylon stockings that would have made a novel but expensive present for a devoted husband to lay at the feet of the little woman. And though the little woman no longer had to worry about finding coupons for a new frock to wear when the dinner things were washed up on Christmas day she still had to worry about finding the thirty shillings to pay for the frock. Life may have started getting a little easier since the war ended, but it wasn't too easy even now.

The spirit of peace and goodwill to all men that should have seeped into every heart once the first Christmas card appeared in the shops had taken an early setback in my home and on the ward where I worked. When the children got to know that Christmas Day was on a Thursday that year and Mummy worked on Thursdays, they rushed to tell Daddy who immediately went off the idea of Mummy going out to work at all. I could go back after Christmas, he said, but how was the cockerel we had been fattening up for the last six months ever to get brown if I wasn't there to baste it? And how were the mince pies and sausage rolls ever to get into the oven if the head-cook-and-kitchen-maid combined was working away instead of carrying out her wifely duties in the kitchen? He asked a great many more questions in the same querulous vein.

Husbands of part-time nurses everywhere were asking the same question. They were quick to point out that teachers and shop assistants, the women who worked in the factory down the road and shorthand typists all had Christmas off, so why did nurses have to be so different and go on working as if it was the same as any ordinary time? The excuses we made about the patients needing looking after as much at

Christmas as at any other time sounded inadequate even to our ears.

In the end it was left to the ward sisters to negotiate a settlement that would silence the husbands of the part-timers, heal the hard-done by feelings of the full-timers and still ensure that the patients got their slice of turkey in as festive an atmosphere as possible. The fact that they were spending Christmas in hospital often meant that they were in no fit state to pull crackers and wishbones. The fit ones went home for Christmas, if they had a home to go to.

The settlements the sisters negotiated involved a lot of hard bargaining. One part-timer could have Christmas Day off so long as she undertook to work on Christmas Eve and Boxing Day; another part-timer who had no children to hang up stockings for was prevailed upon to work on Christmas Day with promises of New Year's Eve and even New Year's Day to compensate. The compromises that had to be made engendered as much ill-feeling as good will. The poor old cockerel that was living out its last days behind chicken wire was never as henpecked as the husband who had to be taught how to mix the ingredients to stuff it with.

Because of the freezing cold November we had shivered through, there were coal fires blazing in almost every hearth and smoke belching blackly from as many chimneys. The smoke blended with the annual pea-souper fog and formed a smog which we lost ourselves in whenever we set foot outside the house. Those who had no urgent reason to go out stayed in until it became easier for them to see a hand in front of their face. The postman and the milkman stayed at home after they found themselves leaving pintas on the wrong doorstep or dropping letters into the wrong boxes. The bus drivers abandoned their vehicles after they had driven twice up a cul-de-sac instead of turning left into the High Street. The world went suddenly quiet – at least the part of the world that was enshrouded with smog.

People like nurses, and others who didn't necessarily have to drive anything or even ride in anything to get to work went to work, taking a terrible time to get there. We wrapped scarves round our mouths and noses, leaving only our bleary eyes exposed like some ghastly Eastern promise, or we bought ready-made masks which were sold at grossly inflated prices by chemists glad of the chance to drum up a bit of extra trade before Christmas. They were already right out of tins of talc and tablets of fancy soap. There had been a run on the soap. Though it had been off the ration for a couple of years it was still a luxury gift for a much-loved mother or a specially cherished girlfriend. It made a nice change from the writing paper everybody gave to everybody while the soap was rationed.

The first morning I stumbled into work after colliding with every brick wall that stood in my path, I was surprised to find Lynch already there. She lived in one of the Nissen huts on a site a fairly long bus ride away from the hospital. The Nissen huts were wartime relics that had been converted into desperately needed peacetime homes. Lynch said it was a terrible thing to have to live in one. They had corrugated roofs that made the pitter-patter of raindrops sound like giant hailstones, and walls down which the condensation ran in streams. Some even had a coke stove with a chimney that bored its way through the living room ceiling. She said it was like being in the army except for the privileges she got from not being in the army. One of the privileges was her handsome Irish husband. That they were so happy with each other almost made up for having to live in a Nissen hut, but the damp was terribly bad for the little boy's chest, Lynch said.

'How on earth did you manage to get in before me?' I asked her, ashamed at straggling in behind the auxiliary when I should have been there first, setting a good example.

'I expect it was because I came by bus and you didn't,' she said tactfully, knowing how important it was for me to set a good example.

'But there aren't any buses running,' I protested. 'At least, there weren't any running where I live.' I felt aggrieved that some should run while others stood idle in the depot. It added more confusion to the confusion we had already been thrown into by the smog. Lynch rushed in to defend herself against a charge of monopolizing the bus service.

'There was only one running from where I live,' she said, sensing my aggrievement, 'and even that one didn't run. We had to walk in front of it carrying torches to show the driver the way. It was hysterical. We were doing fine until we got halfway down the hill then we led him into the cemetery when we should have gone straight on. None of us knew we were in the cemetery until somebody noticed this tombstone thing right in front of the front wheels. The driver was furious with us. He had to reverse for miles. He used a lot of bad language while he was reversing. You'd never have thought we were in a holy place like a cemetery, and he wasn't a bit grateful to us for showing him the way with our torches.' She sounded very indignant at man's ingratitude to torch bearers.

'But I still don't quite see how you managed to get in before me,' I said after I had finished laughing about the tombstone.

'Well, I've already told you,' said Lynch, sounding surprised at my obtuseness. 'I came by bus and you had to walk.' I thought it better not to press her any further but the way I saw it if the passengers had to walk in front of the bus the bus could only have been travelling at a walking pace, which wouldn't have quickened the journey at all; in fact, the time spent going into and backing out of the cemetery must have added several minutes to the track record. There had to be another explanation but I never got it. There were times when Lynch saw things in a different way from me. It probably had something to do with her being Irish. I worked with an Irish girl while I was doing my training and she had her own way of looking at things, which endeared her even more to me.

Brown came in exceptionally late on one of the smoggy mornings. She had a silly look on her face and, when we asked her what had delayed her so much, she tried to sound angry.

'Somebody moved the sign post in the night,' she said.

'Which sign post?' we asked.

'The one at the bottom of the hill,' she fumed. 'They turned the bloody thing round so that all the arms were facing the wrong way. I walked on down to the RAF camp before I realized where I was.'

We learned later that she hadn't just walked down as far as the RAF camp, she had walked right into it, mistaking its fog-shrouded gates for the hospital gates. The airman on sentry duty had asked a lot of questions before he requested an escort to march her back up the road. It had taken Brown and the escort a long time to feel their way back to the hospital. He was a nice sort of fellow she said, older than most of the airmen who strolled up and down the High Street in the evenings making false promises to the local girls. He was due out of the RAF in a couple of years' time and was already planning to buy a little pub somewhere. He hadn't got a wife or any other complications to wash the glasses for him. Brown quite liked the idea of drawing her own pints from the wood. She didn't mind waiting for a couple of years. She had waited a long time already.

Bailey had her own smog story to tell. She had gone to the pictures the evening before with the young man she met at the West Indian club not far from the hospital. When she told us that they hadn't seen much of the film we nudged each other knowingly. It wasn't like that at all, she said haughtily. She and the young man were very respectable; they had only sat in the back row because that was where the usherette had put them. The reason they hadn't seen much of the film was because the smog had seeped into the cinema and obscured their view of the screen. After they had stood strictly to attention right through 'God Save the Queen', she and her respectable young man found their way back to his little car and drove off with the honourable intention of getting back to the hospital at a respectable time. Unfortunately nothing had gone right for them –

or fortunately everything had gone wrong for them, depending on which way you looked at it. The young man had driven round and round the first roundabout, taken a wrong exit and finished up going in the opposite direction altogether from the hospital. Bailey had a faraway look in her eyes when she told us how well they had got to know each other while they were going round and round the roundabout. Nothing would have worked out nearly as well for them if they had only gone round it once and taken the proper exit. Being respectable was sometimes a hindrance to getting to know somebody very well, and a smoggy night was just what they needed to get things going for them.

'But won't you have to go to the Matron for being in late?' I asked her, remembering the days when ten o'clock was deadline, fog or no fog; a minute later and we would be sweating outside the Matron's office waiting to be snarled at by her dog.

'Good Lord no,' said Bailey, laughing at me and my old-fashioned ideas. 'Why on earth should I have to go to her? I'm nearly nineteen, I can please myself when I come in.' I gathered that the sins the student nurses committed no longer had to be recorded in the lodgeman's register. They were allowed to go unhindered up the drive. They weren't even thought of as sins any more.

'The Sanatorium has to send transport down to the town to pick up nurses who have missed the last bus,' said Brown, knowing that I would recall the days when we had to walk a long way down dark lanes if we stayed to watch the end of the big picture.

I could hardly believe what she said about sending transport; I didn't want to believe it. It was all too unsettling for me. It was as if somebody had told my mother that she would still get to heaven even if she didn't go to church twice every Sunday. Lynch said she knew exactly how I felt; she had felt the same when they told her that missing Mass occasionally wouldn't inevitably ruin her chances of going to heaven as she had been taught since infant school to believe it would. She agreed with me that changes were all right in small doses, but too many could destroy the foundations. I was already feeling some of my foundations crumbling beneath my feet.

Not all the smog stories were as happy as Brown's and Bailey's. Some were funny, some were sad, some were a little of both. The lady who walked out of Casualty, happy at being told that the leg she thought was broken was only bruised, wasn't nearly as happy when she collided in the smog with an ambulance that was parked outside Casualty, and broke the bruised leg. Being told in Casualty five minutes later that it was only a simple fracture didn't console her at all while she waited for the plaster to be put on. Colliding with a stationary ambulance was as ridiculous as being run over by a hearse. The man in the pub who swore that that had happened to him said it was just as well the hearse was on its way to the cemetery instead of on the way back. The cracking pace at which they returned to base once their solemn duties were over would almost certainly have resulted in his being bundled into the vehicle and back to the cemetery. Nobody in the pub believed him, but, with all the other peculiar things that were happening in the smog, it just might well have been true.

The police were no more amused than the lady with the broken leg when the man they brought in to have his head examined pending further enquiries nipped smartly through a lavatory window and was lost for ever in the smog. The doctor who examined his head said that he had almost certainly fractured his skull, but it would need to be X-rayed to establish the fact beyond all reasonable doubt. The man hadn't waited long enough to have the fact established; he took a chance on the doctor being wrong. Since he didn't turn up at the hospital later, with all the signs of a fractured skull, his faith in a doctor occasionally making mistakes was justified. Although the police were concerned about his skull, they were also concerned about the trail of broken windows he had left behind him in the town that night. There were a lot of windows broken during that murky week. The murk was an excellent cover-up for crime; it was better than a getaway car.

Part Three

Chapter Ten

THE SMOG WENT on. It congested lungs, clogged up bronchial tubes and gave air passages no room to breathe. People who were out of hospital were rushed into one as fast as the ambulance men could find the entrance, and those who were already in hospital got complications that were worse than the things they were originally admitted with. People who had never had a chest complaint in their lives were suddenly becoming chesty, and those who had enjoyed ill health for years with something the doctors all said was only in the mind made fools of the doctors by dying of it.

We pushed oxygen cylinders round the ward and pegged out oxygen tents when the cylinders weren't enough. We charged and recharged our syringes and stuck so many needles into so many bottoms that the time came when there was nowhere left to stick a needle without finding a sore spot caused by the last needle we stuck in. There shouldn't have been any sore spots; we had all been taught that sore spots, like bed sores, were incontrovertible evidence of bad nursing. But we were much too busy to stand at every bedside after every injection tenderly massaging the site of a potential sore spot.

Although poultices were largely things of the past, huge tins of clay-like paste were dragged out of cupboards in the medical room, the paste was hotted up, spread on lint and applied to the patients' chests. It seldom succeeded where an antibiotic had failed.

One of the doctors who regularly visited the ward started having qualms about ordering so many antibiotics for the old ladies. He said that all he was doing was postponing the inevitable by offering another few days of medicated survival. The phrase sounded very grand and none of us was quite sure what it meant, neither were we sure whether withholding the antibiotics would hasten the inevitable, or if the inevitable would happen just as quickly if we went on giving them. It wasn't easy to tell with the elderly; they were too close to death anyway.

Another doctor whom we all knew to be a committed Christian went on ordering the antibiotics despite his unshakeable belief that God had the final say in setting the time and place for the final breath. The same doctor was also known to hold the opinion that God sent the babies – but this, Brown thought, was most unlikely.

'If God sends the babies, then why does He send so many to people who don't want them and none at all to my sister who has yearned for one for years?' she asked us after she heard about the doctor's beliefs. We didn't know. We were in no position to answer such difficult theological riddles. She asked the doctor and even he couldn't give an answer that would satisfy her, so he quickly changed the subject and went on to something easier. Having a belief was one thing, but trying to rationalize it to somebody as argumentative as Brown would have taken far too long. Lynch said she thought the Pope might know the answer, but he was in Rome and not available for questioning. I wasn't sure that even he would have an answer that Brown could understand. I remembered the Roman Catholic lady who came to me for advice when God kept sending her babies that hadn't been specifically ordered. The Pope seemed to be giving her more problems rather than helping her with those she already had.

But in spite of the antibiotics, the oxygen cylinders and the poultices, some of our grannies still died. We were sad to see them go. We felt they might have lived for ever if the smog hadn't come and killed them.

When the last smoggy patch had dispersed, leaving a dull grey wintry sky in its place, there had been quite a few changes on the Female Chronic ward. Among the changes was an empty bed where Mrs Small once ruled.

She died one night keeping the nurses busy while she died. From the time she was admitted she had flatly refused to let anybody give her medications that would have prolonged the inevitable. She had turned down dexadrin and purple hearts which were then the fashionable things for a doctor to prescribe as aids to slimming – later the fashion was blamed for starting the drug addiction that was to cause the doctors so much despair. She turned down offers of heart tablets for her heart condition and offers of stomach powders for her stomach upsets, and finally she turned down offers of antibiotics for the pneumonia that killed her. The reason she gave for turning down the things we offered her was that it would be against her religion to take them. Though none of us believed her, nobody was willing to take a chance on forcing things on to her at the expense of her soul. She died telling the night nurses that it was against her religion to have one of those nasty dirty bedpans; she wanted to be taken to the lavatory where she always went when she wanted to go. She died sitting on the bedpan. The nurses who had sat her on it felt very guilty. It seemed that not only had they spoilt her chances of eternal life by making her do something that was against her religion, they had also murdered her.

When Mrs Small's visitors came to the ward to enquire where the mortuary was, they said that as far as they knew she had never had a religion. She was C of E, of course, but that wasn't exactly a religion, was it? It was just something that everybody was if they weren't RC, which Mrs Small most certainly wasn't, nor anybody else in the family except an old aunt who had gone funny in the head. They said that the only time any of them could remember Mrs Small going to church was the day she married Mr Small and exactly a year to the day later when she buried him. The night nurses were very relieved when we told them; it at least exonerated them from a charge of murder.

Bailey and I went to the funeral to represent the ward. It was quite an occasion. There were three glossy limousines piled high with wreaths and an oak coffin with solid brass handles. A close relative told us that Mrs Small had been paying the man from the insurance company twopence a week for years to ensure that she got a good send off when her time came. She would have expected the best and she had it.

With the bonuses that accrued from the policy, there was enough to pay for the funeral and provide everybody with a sit-down knife and fork tea. A lot sat down to it. The mourners had come from far and wide. The old lady had been in hospital for such a long time that most of them had forgotten she even existed until the telegram came telling them that she existed no longer. They were all in deepest black.

When Sally, who was getting nearer to being a hundred every day, saw what was happening to Mrs Small and one or two of the others she had done battle with on the verandah, she resolutely refused to follow their example. She was determined to live to be a hundred if it was the last thing she did. At the sign of the slightest chill she took to her bed and rapped her stick on the bed table day and night, demanding the things the others were getting to delay their departure. We willingly gave them to her. We poured linctus down her throat, stuck needles into her thin old bottom and even slapped poultices on her chest. We would have hated her to be disappointed at the last minute.

Happily she lived just long enough to be able to boast that she had lived to be a hundred. She would have been extremely upset if she had known she could have lived a year less and still boasted. When the records were scrutinized they showed that she was a hundred and one instead of the straight century she had striven so hard to achieve, and almost driven us mad helping her to achieve. She went out in a blaze of anger. Right to the end she was finding something to argue with everybody about. There was nothing peaceful about Sally's passing.

Brown and the ward sister went to her funeral. They were the only ones there except for the vicar and the undertaker's men. There were no wreaths, just a small spray we had collected for amongst ourselves on the ward. Sally didn't have a family to summon by telegram, and none of her friends had lived even to be a hundred never mind a hundred and one. Not only is it wearing to live so long, it can be a very lonely existence.

Jennie also died during the dreary days, but not of pneumonia or any of the other complications that the smog brought with it. Suddenly she seemed not to want to go on living any longer. Try as Bailey might, she couldn't make the accounts of the films she and her young man went to see interesting enough to interest Jennie. For a while we went on getting her up and strapping her into her chair, but with nothing for her to look at in the ward she sat looking hopelessly into space, just as the chronics had done in the past. Lottie did her best to coax her with spoonsful of this and spoonsful of that and feeding-cups of nourishing drinks but, with all her loving screaming, little of what she offered Jennie went the way it should have gone. None of us was able to do any better. Even Bailey's kind brown hands were pushed away when she pressed Jennie with warm milk and soup.

After Jennie died her mother came out from behind the screens. 'It's better this way, isn't it?' she said, weeping. None of us truly knew. Who does? But talking about it later we decided that it was perhaps better that way. There would have been no future for Jennie, except a life of being lifted from bed to chair and back to bed again, and, even when there were flowers for her to look at from her place on the verandah, there were things that made life unbearable for her sometimes. The blind spot that Brown had talked about didn't always work.

When the smog had gone and Christmas was over we settled down to an eventless routine brightened only by the feverish plans that were being made everywhere for the Coronation celebrations. Any spare time we had was spent making red, white and blue things to prove our loyalty to the new Queen. The Coronation celebrations outdid even the Victory celebrations, though I saw very little of them. We sat in front of the television set most of the day with the curtains closed. It was pouring with rain and the children had both got German measles. Luckily I was on official holiday at the time, so having to be at home while they had German measles didn't make a hole in the pay packet. There were no final demands in the sideboard drawer and the coalman delivered regularly.

Chapter Eleven

WHEN THE THRILLS of the Coronation were over and we were all left with a lot of red, white and blue things we didn't know what to do with, a rumour got around that a man had been admitted to the local isolation hospital with something that might be smallpox. Panic spread rapidly; it was as infectious as the smallpox would have been. People who hadn't previously believed in things like vaccination suddenly found themselves having different thoughts. While smallpox had been just a word, a medieval plague or something you only got if you lived in foreign parts, there seemed no point in the new little baby at home having a scarlet ribbon tied round its arm to protect the scab from being knocked off by a careless passer-by. But smallpox in the fever hospital only a bus ride away was a different matter altogether. It called for immediate action. Soon the roads were blocked with winding trails of parents and children all bound for the nearest doctor's surgery, the welfare clinic or one of the special centres set up for mass vaccination. The doctors quickly ran out of their stocks of vaccine, and the staff at the clinics and centres were quickly run off their feet. There had been nothing like it since the shops ran out of bread.

Dilys brought me the news of the smallpox scare. She rushed in one Tuesday morning dragging her twins behind her.

'Have you heard the news?' she gasped, breathless and dramatic.

'What news?' I asked, giving the children a biscuit each.

'The news about the smallpox,' said Dilys, helping herself to two biscuits. 'It's everywhere. They're dying like flies with it in the fever hospital.' I stood for a moment thinking about the fever hospital. It was very small. It had lost a lot of its usefulness after people stopped dying like flies in it with scarlet fever and diphtheria. There was even talk of turning parts of it into an annexe of the main hospital and sending the geriatrics down there. But that was still only a rumour, as I hoped Dilys's news about the smallpox was.

The reason I was at home on Tuesday instead of at work where my professional duty lay was because the youngest had wakened that morning with earache. I was sorry about the earache, but I wasn't too pleased with her for having it on Tuesday. I was only too aware of the hardship it would cause to those who would have to struggle on at work without me. I remembered how the sister and I had had to struggle on when I first went back to work and Lynch had rung in to say her little boy had got the measles, and how we had had to struggle on without her again when he had an attack of something that nobody seemed able to diagnose. Not being able to diagnose it had made things very hard for Lynch when she eventually returned to work. Reporting back with insufficient evidence that the absence was due to something dire and identifiable gave rise to a lot of suspicion among the other nurses on the ward. If a part-time married nurse or any of her family had to be ill, then for everybody's sake let the illness be one that could be pinned down and labelled. Anything less, and the absentee might just have been absent because she wanted to get the blankets washed while the weather was fine, or have the sitting room papered in time for Christmas. Nurses were a nasty suspicious lot when it came to other nurses having time off that wasn't allowed for in their conditions of service.

When Selina came round earlier that morning to find out why the children hadn't been taken round to her, she had looked at the one with earache and clucked ominously. Having brought up six sons to puberty and beyond she thought she knew all there was to be known about children's ailments.

'It's mastoids,' she said, casting a woeful eye at the woeful sufferer. Being a nurse I knew perfectly well that it wasn't mastoids, but being a mother I knew she was right. I saw in a flash every child I had ever nursed with mastoids. I thought of all those who had died in spite of my nursing, and I remembered others who had gone home with terrible and permanent complications when the mastoids were better. My heart sank like lead until I thought of antibiotics, then it lifted again. Then I looked back into the aching ear, but this time with a professional eye rather than with a mother's biased anxiety.

'Of course it isn't mastoids, it's earache,' I said, giving the youngest a little hug for not having mastoids and for being a good girl and standing still while I looked into her ear.

Selina gave a shrug of weary resignation.

'Oh well, if that's what you want to think then so be it, but you'll see,' she said darkly and went off to take the one who hadn't got earache to school, and also to ring the hospital for me to tell them I wouldn't be in.

I was always grateful to anybody who would ring the hospital for me to tell them I wouldn't be in. It was a task I shirked doing. However genuine the excuse for my absence might be, the nervous way I conveyed it to whoever was taking the message at the other end could only convince them that I was up to my elbows in suds washing the blankets or perched on a ladder tearing paper off the sitting room walls. When the eldest got older she was given the responsibility of breaking the news that I wouldn't be in, unless she was responsible for me not being in, then the youngest was primed word for word on what to say and how to say it to make the excuse sound plausible. Even then there were times when I walked back on the ward knowing that I was under a cloud of suspicion. I hoped the cloud wouldn't be too dense when I got back the following Monday morning. I knew from experience that it would be Monday before I reported on duty again, however devotedly I nursed the earache. It was a constant source of wonder to the full-time nurses how the children of the part-timers managed to do the bulk of their suffering during the days when their mothers should have been at work. It was even more of a mystery to the part-timers how their children could suffer untold agony from Monday to Friday yet, when Saturday dawned, be up at the crack ready to queue outside Saturday morning pictures to watch Flash Gordon, or Roy Rogers doing things on his horse, Trigger, they would have liked to be doing themselves.

'Are you sure about the smallpox?' I asked Dilys while I was getting the warm oil and cotton wool ready for the next application.

'Of course I'm sure,' she said, sounding absolutely certain. 'Ginger, the milkman who delivers down at the fever hospital – you know, the one who's got "cut here" tattooed round his neck – told my mam about it when she was giving him his cup of tea this morning, and she rushed round to tell me. That's why I've rushed round to tell you. He said he'd heard a rumour that a man had been admitted in the night with something that might be smallpox. But you know how these things spread – there could be hundreds in there by now, dying like flies.' I was greatly relieved at the watered-down version of the rumour. One man in the fever hospital with something that might be smallpox sounded a little more hopeful than hundreds dying like flies with it. But I knew that even one suspect would be causing grave anxiety. I could imagine the frantic search that might already be going on to track down the man's contacts. I hoped there wouldn't be too many, especially if the man became a confirmed case instead of merely a suspect. With all that had been done to kill off smallpox it would be sad to see it coming to life again in our own small fever hospital only a bus ride away.

'What do you think I should do about them?' said Dilys, looking at the twins, who were looking at the biscuit tin with avaricious eyes.

'You don't need to do anything about them,' I said putting the biscuit tin away to indicate that there were no more forthcoming. 'They've both been vaccinated, haven't they?'

A trace of embarrassment crossed Dilys's face.

'As a matter of fact, they haven't,' she said, the embarrassment in her face turning to a small note of defiance in her voice. 'My dad wouldn't let us have them done. He says he can show you statistics to prove that there are as many children that die of being vaccinated as die of smallpox. He doesn't believe in things like vaccination. He says it's going against nature.' I knew nothing at all about statistics but I was almost sure there would be enough to prove that more children, and adults too, died of smallpox than would ever die of being vaccinated. But it was no time to be troubling Dilys with statistics, even if I could have come up with any.

'Get them done,' I said firmly. Dilys rushed off to join the queue that was snaking its way up the hill.

I didn't have to join the queue. I had the same feelings about vaccination as I did about baptism. If there were any benefits to be derived from either, I considered it my duty as their mother to see that my children became eligible for the benefits with as little delay as possible. I took them to church and wiped away a tear while the parson christened them, and I took them to the doctor and steadfastly refused to look while he vaccinated them. If by some dreadful mischance the parson had dropped them in the font and drowned them, or they had suffered some awful and permanent damage from being vaccinated, I would have been destroyed but not perhaps as guilt-ridden as I would have been if they had gone to the Devil at some later date, or been scarred for life by smallpox, because I had neglected to take the necessary steps to avert either tragedy. But that may have been just my way of looking at things because I was a nurse. Whether I would have been influenced by the propaganda that was soon to stir up feelings against such things as vaccination and immunization would be hard to tell, though I would have joined any queue that would have stopped the children going blue in the face when they had whooping cough.

The man in the fever hospital didn't have smallpox after all. Dilys's dad was very angry with me for putting daft ideas in his daughter's head. He came round and shook his fist at me and threatened what he would do if I didn't stop poking my nose into other people's business. He said a few things in Welsh that I didn't understand and went off still shaking his fist.

After he had gone I sat and had a cup of tea to steady my nerves and told myself that, if the man in the fever hospital had turned out to have smallpox instead of being just a suspect, Dilys's dad might have been grateful to me for reducing his grandchildren's chances of catching it, unless of course they had borne out his statistical evidence and been made worse instead of better by the vaccination. It wasn't always easy to make the right decisions for other people, especially when the decisions involved their children. It wasn't always easy to make the right decisions about one's own children; the only thing to work on, with them, was whatever resulted from hours and hours of tossing and turning in the night trying to reach a decision.

The smallpox scare soon died down and people stopped having their babies vaccinated, saying they didn't believe in it and that it wasn't necessary now that there was no danger of them catching smallpox anyway. It was often hard for them to understand that the reason their children were in less danger of catching smallpox was because somebody had come up with the idea of vaccinating them against it. If the idea was allowed to go to waste the danger of catching smallpox would be with us again. But that was propaganda that men like Dilys's dad outwitted with their statistics.

We used our summer annual leave after the Coronation to move out of the tiny terraced house into one that was slightly larger and only unilaterally attached to the house next to it. The move took us a notch or two up the social scale. The day had still to dawn when vast sums of money were spent on turning tiny terraced houses into highly desirable town dwellings. A terraced house was a terraced house, a semi had more class.

The move also meant that we acquired a cooker that looked the same as everybody else's cooker, a garden gate of our own and a path that led exclusively to our front door instead of having to be shared with the neighbours as we had shared the pig bin. The cooker, the gate and the exclusive use of the path were terribly exciting for me at first. I switched the oven on and off and swung the garden gate forwards and backwards until it almost fell of its hinges. I felt about them as the children felt about the new toys they had for Christmas and birthdays. The novelty lasted for as short a time.

We had to leave the pullets behind when we moved. There was no room for them in our neat new garden. The children were sad at leaving them behind: they had watched them grow from chickens and looked on them as part of the family. We offered them to our old land-lord as sitting tenants, and he kindly invited us to drop in and see them if we were ever in the neighbourhood. We never dropped in. We abandoned the pullets to their fate and bought the children a goldfish to mend their broken hearts.

We had to leave Selina behind as well. Though the house we were moving to was only on the other side of the town her bunions would never have allowed her to trudge across twice a day to be a grandma to the children when I wasn't there. Leaving her behind was as painful and gave us more problems than leaving the pullets behind. We could buy an egg from the grocer's whenever we needed one, and we still had a few left in the preserving jar, but getting another Selina wasn't easy. She had been a very special person: always at hand when I needed her and always with a ready hand to chastise the children if she thought they needed it. But however often the children came home complaining that Selina had smacked them on a place specially padded for smacking they were always ready to go back the next day to eat the sticky buns she buttered for them. She mingled discipline with kindness in exactly the right proportions which I seldom did. I was either too heavy-handed with the discipline or over-indulgent with the buns. Getting the proportions right takes endless patience and a fund of wisdom, qualities which are usually only fully developed after the mother becomes a grandmother, when the mixture is called 'spoiling the grandchildren'.

We had used the summer holiday for moving house partly because if I had taken special leave it would have upset the staffing arrangements on the ward, and partly because if we had both taken special leave it would have upset the financial arrangements at home. Using the summer holiday for moving meant that we didn't get a proper holiday that year. This didn't trouble any of us too much; we had had a proper holiday the year before, and it hadn't been a holiday at all. Even the children looked back on it and remembered only the bad parts. There hadn't been any good parts for them to remember.

Until then we had spent all our going-away holidays with my parents. It pleased my parents, made a nice change for the children and – the greatest boon of all – except for fares to pay and sundries to buy, it was free. But suddenly, the year before we moved, we had started to get itchy feet. We needed to stretch our wings and find fresh fields and pastures new. The endless stretches of fields and pastures round my father's smallholding had begun to pall.

When I told Selina about our urge to travel, she at once suggested that we should go to a little place where she and her husband always went when they got itchy feet, which was every summer when his works shut down for a week. It was the seaside, she said, and just what the children needed to set them up for the winter. For the modest sum of three pounds a week, adults in season, children half-price, we could count on getting three home-cooked meals a day, eaten in a homely atmosphere, with hot and cold running water thrown in at no extra cost. It was also no more than an hour's journey by train from London.

It rained heavily on the morning we set out for our first proper holiday *en famille*. It was still raining when we got to the seaside. We travelled wetly around looking for the select guest house to which we had sent the stamped addressed envelope and five shillings deposit as security against us changing our minds at the last minute. None of the bedraggled people we saw in the almost deserted town had ever heard of the select guest house, neither had they heard of the street it was in; but, intrepid travellers that we were we eventually came upon it. It was not the Ritz – but it was very homely.

Our landlady was the proud owner of a cuckoo clock and four dogs. The cuckoo clock hung from a hook immediately outside our family-sized room. Unlike most cuckoo clocks it was the genuine Black Forest article and in perfect working order. At regular intervals there came a whirring noise and a little wooden bird sprang out of its little wooden chalet to announce the time with a sprightly eagerness that was charming at first, irritating after the first hour or two and quite mind-bending after several hours of lying in wide-eyed anticipation of its next announcement. It obviously didn't speak English; it took no notice when my husband addressed it in a few well-chosen words.

The dogs were small hairy creatures. They were nasty, snappy little dogs. They hated children and disliked strangers. The children were children and we were all strangers. We had embarrassing confrontations whenever we went to the running hot and cold water, which was far enough away from the family-sized room to give the dogs plenty of scope for attack. Each child had to be accompanied by an adult before it would set foot on the landing.

We wandered for a long time in the rain before we came across the sea. The children were very disappointed in it. They had expected waves and white horses, sea shells and sand castles, and maybe even a palm tree or two waving gently in the balmy breeze. The sea that lay beyond the weather-beaten old parapet we leaned perilously over was nothing like that: in the gloom that faced us we could faintly discern a ripple of water that appeared to be lapping the edge of a wide expanse of black mud.

My husband looked accusingly at me.

'Well, there it is,' he said, as if I had put it there. 'There's your sea. That's what we've been saving up for ever since Christmas. I kept telling you we should have gone to your mother's like we always do.' He had kept telling me nothing of the sort. He had been as keen on coming to the seaside as I was. He had even gone out and bought swimming trunks for himself and a bucket and spade for the children. They were still in the suitcase in their original wrappings.

It kept on raining. We sat squabbling and bickering under the shelters on the esplanade. When we hinted to our landlady that since there was nothing we could do outside we might be allowed to stay in, she was aghast at the idea. She reminded us in no uncertain terms that the Urban District Council had spent a great deal of money to provide shelters for visitors to sit under when it rained. It rained a lot in that particular area, and if she had her paying guests running in and out at every drop she wouldn't know where she was, now would she? We agreed that she wouldn't, then hurried off before she set the dogs on us.

It stopped raining on Saturday. The sun shone and the sky dazzled us with its blueness. We stood for a moment looking over the parapet on our way to the station, but we couldn't linger in case we missed our train. We got home hot and tired from the heat of an August day. The next morning we set out early and went to the Lido not a mile from where we lived and came home in the evening as red as beetroots.

It took us a day or two to settle down after the holiday. The children wanted chips and bottles of ketchup with everything and none of us slept too well. We missed being kept awake by the cuckoo clock.

When we took Selina the stick of rock we'd brought back for her from the seaside she asked us what the holiday was like. We said it was marvellous and thanked her for recommending the place to us, but when we touched lightly on the weather she looked at us in astonishment.

'You don't go there for the weather,' she said, sounding as astonished as she looked. 'You go for the amusement arcade further up the road. It's covered in and you could have sat in there all day doing your knitting or reading a book while the children played on the dodgem cars and the slot machines. You wouldn't have known whether it was raining or not outside.' It seemed we had made a terrible hash of our first proper holiday.

But whatever else the week by the sea did for us – or didn't do for us – at least it satisfied our urge for travel. We were quite content the next year to use the holiday time for moving house and the holiday money to put down as a deposit on the new cooker though when the moving was finished and it was time for me to go back to work, I still hadn't found a replacement for Selina. All I had found was somebody who would take the children to school for me in the mornings and let them quarrel with her own children until I collected them in the afternoon. I had still to solve the problem of all the school holidays that stretched ahead. I solved it while I was giving my husband his supper one evening.

Chapter Twelve

Because the war had dragged on for years, instead of ending in months as the optimists predicted it would, great gaps began to appear in the structure of our health service: not the pie-in-the-sky Health Service that rashly promised to make illness an exciting free adventure instead of a painfully expensive luxury, but the old health service that had been with us for as long as any of us could remember and for as long again before that.

The existing hospitals were inadequate to take the added weight of wartime patients. There were never enough beds to go round. As well as the more dramatic casualties, there were still the run-of-the-mill patients with run-of-the-mill complaints. Urgent plans were soon having to be drawn up to find ways of accommodating the overspill. The plans took shape almost overnight and became basic wooden huts, originally intended as temporary arrangements to tide us over until the war was over when lots of lovely new hospitals could be built. But lots of lovely new hospitals needed lots of lovely old money, and even when the war was over better uses could be found for whatever money there was than throwing it away on frivolous indulgences like hospitals. The wooden huts stayed to become a shabby reflection of the priorities of those whose business it was to apportion the nation's wealth.

The monstrous Victorian hospitals also stayed, with their cockroach-infested kitchens and their gloomy corridors overhung with naked plumbing arrangements that gave them the look of medieval torture chambers rather than vital links from one part of a hospital to the other. Taking children down one of the corridors could turn the walk into a nightmare that would stay in their subconscious dreams for ever. Putting a child in a lift that threatened to shudder to a stop somewhere between the first and second floors was no encouragement to them to: 'Stop crying, do, before the doctor hears you and says what a baby you are.' Even strong men were made cowards by the grimness of the waiting rooms they had to sit in until it was their turn to be seen by their own particular consultant.

But it was a long time before a bit of wet cement got slapped on a brick or a turf was eased out of the ground by a Very Important Person or a less important local dignitary, and a board was put up on the site telling the town that with a bit of luck their new hospital would be completed several years hence. By the side of the board there was usually a huge mock thermometer with mock mercury that rose in proportion to the amount of money that had been raised at the last jumble sale, or extorted from people at the Christmas bazaar.

The buildings rose as slowly as the mercury. Strikes had become fashionable among the workers. That it was a hospital they were working on didn't stop them from downing tools to a man when the call for 'everybody out' came over the Tannoy system. The hospital could wait until the union meeting was over, the industrial dispute ended or the labour problems were solved. Strikes were known by many different names but none of the names made them smell any sweeter. Each strike crippled the post-war building programme more than the last one had.

And in the meantime the wooden huts began to deteriorate. After many more years of wear and tear than they had ever been intended to take, most of them were in urgent need of a facelift, or even a bit of cosmetic surgery to keep them looking young for a few more years. The facelifts took time to complete, and while they were being done the huts had to be emptied to leave room for the workers to work or have their tea breaks in comfort.

When it was the turn of the hut I worked in to get its face lifted, the Matron invited Lynch, Brown and me to go to the office for a little chat. Bailey and the ward sister were not invited. They had already been told what was in store for them. Being full-time and resident gave them less say in the shaping of their destinies. Their destinies were still being shaped for them by the system, though not as rigorously as mine was shaped for me when I was full-time and resident. At least they were allowed to come in when they liked at night without having to sweat outside the office in the morning.

Being part-time and married gave Lynch and me the right to choose what hours we would work. Brown, though not married, was neither a nurse in training nor resident, so she could claim one or two privileges that being married would have entitled her to. Changing her duties was one of the pre-marital privileges she claimed; whether there were any more we didn't know. If there were, she never mentioned them to us, though she occasionally came on duty in the morning looking like a cat who has been fed cream instead of skimmed milk. The morning look usually coincided with a previous evening spent with her airman, but whether that was anything but sheer coincidence could only be guessed at.

The Matron began the chat by asking Lynch how her little boy was, went on to ask me how my little daughters were and when she had enquired kindly after Brown's arches she told us why we were there. The patients on the ward where we worked were to be moved down to one of the empty wards at the fever hospital – not just for the duration of the facelift but permanently, thus leaving more wards in the main hospital available for acute cases. Unless we were utterly opposed to the idea she intended sending us down to the fever hospital with the patients. She looked at us and waited for us to tell her if we were utterly opposed to the idea. We were not, but we had certain amendments to make to it.

The rumours about turning part of the fever hospital into an annexe for geriatrics had been in circulation long enough for us to have thought about it and decided whether we would be opposed to going down there or not. I had spent sleepless nights wondering how I could turn any move I might make to my own advantage. After much weary tossing I had thought of a scheme whereby the children would have a mother whenever they needed one during the day and hopefully wouldn't even notice that she had forsaken them in the night. With nobody like Selina to stand in as grandma for them, night duty seemed the perfect solution to the problem of school holidays. It would ensure that I was somewhere around the house even if I was snatching forty winks while they were killing each other in the garden.

Working nine to three-thirty from Monday to Friday had meant that I was never there when they went to school in the morning, nor there when they came home, clamouring for a mini-meal to sustain them until they clamoured for their tea. Doing the later hours of two in the afternoon to eight in the evening would give them the wave to school in the morning, but they would have to eat mini-meal and even tea with no mother there to dispense either. If I worked the later hours, as well as missing out on the mini-meal and the egg and chips at tea time, I would not be there to hear their prayers before I tucked them up at bedtime. Saying their prayers was a nightly ritual that the children valued greatly, not merely for the spiritual rewards they were promised if they said them regularly, but because by saying them regularly they gained a few minutes of extra time before the light was put out or the final good night said. The length of the prayers varied with the prevailing climatic conditions. They could go on and on seemingly endlessly, or be cut short almost before they began.

On summer evenings, when the noonday sun had warmed the bedrooms and the lengthening shadows were pleasant enough to make intimate little chats with Our Father which art in Heaven a charming way of ending the day, I sat on each child's bed in turn and listened to the chat with an attentive ear. I curbed any tendency to gabble and insisted that God bless Mummy – and Daddy, too, of course – should be said with suffi-cient feeling to make the plea rise heavenwards and be taken note of by whoever was up there listening. I allowed mention to be made of all creatures great and small, not forgetting Grandad's horse which had met its end in the gorse bushes a long time ago, and the goldfish which was found floating on its back one morning. I sat in reverent silence while intercession was made for best friends, favourite teachers and everybody who had passed, however briefly, through the children's life. I even threw in a few names on my own account of those who had trespassed against me during the day. The punishments I begged for them were mercifully withheld by the One from whom I was begging the favours.

But in the wintertime, when the breath froze on the windowpanes and the blankets grew damp with condensation, the praying time was severely cut. God bless Mummy etcetera had to be speeded up so that Mummy could be back watching her favourite programme on television in front of the sitting room fire with as much dispatch as possible. A cold winter's night was no time to be pleading for the souls of dead goldfish. When the north wind howled and the snow fell, the final Amen came sooner.

But whether the prayers were said at funereal speed or gabbled with irreverent haste it was unthinkable that I shouldn't be there to hear them, at least until the children were old enough to want to pray in silence. However good a daddy was for throwing rubber ducks at from the bath, prayers demanded a mother's listening ear. Going on night duty was the only way I could think of to combine the wave to school in the morning, the welcome home in the afternoon and the listening ear at prayer time.

'What do you think of the idea of me going on night duty?' I said to my husband one evening while I was buttering him up with all the favourite things he liked for his supper. 'The Matron lets the part-timers do three or four nights a week, and even if I had to do alternate weekends you'd be here on Saturday and Sunday to keep the children quiet while I was in bed. You could even cook their dinner.' I added the last sentence without much hope. His aversion to wearing a pinny was as strong as ever. It would be a long time before he cooked anything more venturesome than a tin of baked beans if I hadn't got everything ready just to lay on the table before I went off to bed.

He spooned more treacle on to his pudding. Treacle pudding was one of his favourite things.

'And when would you sleep if I wasn't here and the children weren't at school?' he asked.

I brushed aside the question as airily as he had brushed aside the suggestion that he should cook a full-scale meal for the children. Sleep would be no problem at all, I assured him. Sleep would be fitted in easily once I got things organized.

I knew I was lying. I had heard other part-time night nurses talking in the locker room. Some of them got hardly any sleep at all when their children were off school, and not enough when they were at school, with all the other things that had to be fitted in. But it wasn't the moment to be dwelling on the drawbacks of night duty. I went into all the advantages until, sweetened with treacle, he agreed that it would be a most advantageous thing for me to go on night duty.

Selina had told me one way of getting a man to agree to anything; I had used the pudding to get my man to agree to something and Lynch did it in a different way altogether.

When I told them at work that if we moved down to the fever hospital I was going to ask the Matron if I could go on night duty, Brown said she wouldn't mind going on nights herself. She was due for a change and the airman who made her come on duty looking so happy did much of what he did in the RAF during the night. She would look happy even more often if they saw more of each other.

Lynch listened and looked thoughtful while we were talking about it, then she went home to persuade her husband that going on nights would solve all their problems as well. The little boy would be leaving the nursery school soon and would need a mother to cling to screaming when the doors of big school opened to swallow him up; he would also need her there to tell her what a lovely day he'd had when he was let loose again in the afternoon.

Her husband wasn't too keen at first on the idea of her rushing out to go to work just when she should have been getting herself in the mood for snuggling up to him in the Nissen hut. But Lynch had snuggled up to him to such good purpose that night that by the morning he had quite come round to the idea. Lynch said that her way of getting a man to agree to anything was far nicer than Selina's or even mine; hers had mutual benefits, especially if you weren't too fond of treacle pudding yourself.

We chose Brown to be spokeswoman and tell the Matron about our plan to go on nights. Lynch excused herself on the grounds that she was shy in front of people like the Matron and, though I was never lost for words when there was nothing to be said, I wasn't good at coming to the point and putting things in nutshells. Brown was good at both. She planted her feet painfully in front of the Matron's desk and spoke. When she had finished, the Matron looked at the three of us and smiled. It was a smile of relief. She told us that the nurses down at the fever hospital had all been there for a long time, and it would be unfair to expect them to change their hours to suit the changing circumstances. More staff would be needed for night duty; she would be very happy for us to fill the gap. And that was that. I was to become a part-time night nurse instead of a part-time day nurse.

The Matron had one small amendment of her own to make. 'Working down at the fever hospital may mean that you could be called upon to go on to one of the infectious diseases wards that are still in use, but only if they became grossly understaffed and there was an epidemic of something that required more nurses to be sent down there. Would any of you have any objections to working on the infectious diseases wards?' She looked at us. Brown said she wouldn't; she had already worked in a fever hospital, though she wasn't fever trained, and had no reason to object. Lynch said she wouldn't mind if we didn't and so long as she didn't give her little boy any of the things she nursed in the fever wards. The Matron smiled kindly at her and assured her that, if she kept to the rules, there would be no danger of that. Then she looked at me. I could see no reason either to object. As far as I could tell, infectious diseases were no longer of much importance. The few that still went round the schools were almost always nursed at home, with the family doctor calling in to renew the free prescriptions for whatever antibiotic was needed to stop any complications, or to clear up the complications if they arose. Only the most acutely complicated were admitted to hospital, and it wasn't to be expected that there would be enough of them to warrant extra staff being sent down to the isolation wards. I was quite happy to say I wouldn't mind going if the need arose. None of us could have foreseen the magnitude of the epidemic that was soon to fill the fever hospitals and have calls going out for extra staff to cope with it.

When we left the office it had been decided that Lynch and I should work seven nights a fortnight – three one week and four the next, the nights to run conjointly, taking in alternate week-ends. The thought of having seven clear nights – and days – at home with my family made the conditions seem Utopian to me. As it turned out, they were not nearly as Utopian as I thought they would be.

Lynch saw farther ahead than I did. 'God,' she said when we got outside. 'I hope it's as good as it sounds. It's too easy; there has to be snags in it somewhere.' She was right: there were.

The move to the geriatric annexe of the fever hospital took longer than anybody had imagined it would. The delay was due mainly to the resistance put up by the grannies against any form of change. Telling them that they were going to be put into an ambulance and whisked off down to the fever hospital caused them as much anguish as if we were begging them to board a plane and fly to the other end of the world. Not only did we have to coax and cajole them into letting us pack their lemon and barley water and sponge bags, we had to remind them that the fever hospital was only a stone's throw down the road and not a million miles away where their visitors would never find them again. Even those who didn't get any visitors knew that there was less chance of a long-lost cousin locating them at the fever hospital down the lane than in the infirmary which was right on the bus route. (Those who had lived in the town all their lives refused to follow current fashion and call the place they were in a hospital. An infirmary it had been since the day it was built, and an infirmary it would always be for them. They would have no fancy names for the grim old building where they had sat waiting sadly for a dear husband or a precious child to die, or where they had watched their parents die too long ago for the year of their death to be recalled.)

The fact that it was the fever hospital they were being moved to only added to their distress. They knew all about the fever hospital: it was the nasty place down the lane that had once been full of people with fevers. Almost all of them could tell heart-rending stories of the time when one, two or even all of their many children had been patients in there, with scarlet fever or diphtheria. If the children were lucky enough to survive the scarlet fever, they often went home with weak hearts, damaged kidneys or some other complication that would stay with them for life. If they were lucky enough to survive the diphtheria they bore the scar for ever of the gash the doctor had had to make in their throats to help them to breathe again.

One of our grannies claimed boastfully that each of her ten children had had its throat cut by a doctor before it was out of its cradle. She claimed just as boastfully that she was the carrier who had given the children diphtheria. She then tearfully told us that she had spent ten of the best years of her life within the walls of the fever hospital because she was a carrier. When we grilled her to get at the truth, she finally broke down and confessed that it may have been ten months, or even a paltry ten weeks, but however long it was she was unshaken in her belief that whatever had kept her there was still there, waiting to strike again the moment her wheelchair crossed the threshold. If the fever hospital had been the point from which the Black Death or the Great Plague had originated it could hardly have struck more fear in the hearts of our grannies who were being asked to spend their few remaining years down there.

One or two of them went to the extremes of almost dying rather than have to suffer the upheaval. Or so it seemed. Whether it was because their resistance had been lowered by the stresses they were having to endure, or because it was wintertime and cold and damp and miserable, we didn't know, but one by one they caught chills, sprang temperatures on us, complained of chest pains, tummy pains and an assortment of things that hurt them though they weren't exactly sure where they hurt. The doctor went over their chests with his stethoscope, ordered antibiotics and put off the moving day again. Wheeling a ninety-year-old down a draughty corridor and out to a waiting ambulance after the night nurse had reported she had sneezed even once in the night could turn the sneeze into something an antibiotic might not be able to cure. It was much longer than had been expected before the doctor hung his stethoscope round his neck, crossed his fingers and said that as far as he could judge the chosen people were ready for the exodus. One by one we loaded them into the ambulances. It was a trying day for all of us.

The fever hospital was a huddle of low grey buildings, most of which had been standing at the end of the lane for a long time. There were three twenty-bedded open wards that were even older than most of our grannies, and one that was outstandingly new: it had never been used since the day it was built in anticipation of an epidemic of something which everybody hoped would never happen. There were also two blocks of single-bedded cubicle wards, a hot and steamy laundry and a chilly mortuary. Between the laundry and the mortuary was the original nurses' home, kept warm by its neighbour on one side and haunted, it was said, by the ghosts of the occupants of the other side. Standing aloof from the rest of the huddle, as if ashamed of being associated with such antiquity, was a new and very modern nurses' home, which had been added when the old one started crumbling with age. A mere facelift wouldn't have been enough to stop the resident nurses in the old home from disappearing under a ton of debris if a force eight gale had sprung up and stayed for more than a day. Such an incident would have brought down the wrath of the various trades unions concerned with making sure that things like that didn't happen to nurses. The bit of wet cement had been slapped on a brick before anything so awful happened.

We unpacked the grannies, their lemon and barley water and their sponge bags and spent a great deal of time arranging and rearranging them in beds that would separate the more warring factions among them. Putting Granny Sweetman next to old Mrs Love, for example, would have turned the ward into Bedlam every time they disagreed over something: neither of them lived up to the promise of their name. But separating them wasn't easy either: most of them liked being next to the ones they hated. A battle a day went a long way towards keeping the doctor away, except for his routine visits. Fighting kept them fit. Far fewer of them died with apoplexy brought on by rage than slipped away quietly through having nothing to aggravate them into staying alive.

But soon they had a cross to bear which drew them together in a united front against us and against whoever had designed the ward they were on. When we told them that there was no verandah for them to sit on they mumbled and grumbled and became very cross indeed. That none of them had ever wanted to sit on the verandah when there was one made no difference at all. The ward soon rang with friendly exchanges of unfriendly criticisms of those who were responsible for the deprivation. Even Granny Sweetman and old Mrs Love began throwing mint humbugs at each other across the intervening beds and a truce, however temporary, was declared.

When the move down to the fever hospital was completed and most of our patients had forgotten they had ever been anywhere else, I took part of my annual leave to get ready for the changeover from days to nights. I spent most of it sitting by my father's bed in a hospital, watching him die.

Part Four

Chapter Thirteen

BEING TOLD BY my mother only the day before I left home to be a nurse that I didn't belong to her, or to my father either, and wasn't at all the girl I had always thought I was, caused me fewer emotional hang-ups than a psychiatrist looking for emotional hang-ups would have expected to find. I had stood for a moment swept by a wave of passionate weeping brought on by romantic images of my poor young natural mother being cruelly deserted by my handsome hero of a natural father, then I had put them both behind me and gone back to being what I had always been – the daughter of a father and mother who had fostered me with love almost since the day I was born, and with no reward for their fostering except for the little pleasure I might have brought them. I wasted no time trying to trace my forebears, and only once took any steps to seek out the place of my birth. Even that was a waste of time, since it was no longer there when I found it; it had been one of the casualties when the Battle of Britain was fought over London. After that I only occasionally gave my natural parents a thought, fleetingly wondering if they were still alive and if so whether they ever thought about me. Living in the past is something which only the old should indulge in, or writers seeking material for their books.

When the telegram arrived telling me that my father was dying, I read it twice through tears, did enough cooking to ensure that my family wouldn't starve while I was away, enough washing to keep them smelling sweet until I got back, and went off alone to the depths of Lincolnshire.

My mother looked at me in bewilderment when I walked through the door.

'Whatever brings you here at this time of night?' she asked.

It was the middle of the afternoon and my turn to look bewildered.

'You sent me a telegram,' I reminded her. She shook her head.

'Nay, that I never did,' she said firmly. 'I don't hold with things like telegrams. They bring nothing but bad news. You can ask your father, he'll tell you the same.'

'Where is he?' I asked her, thinking that he might still be upstairs in the double bed they had shared for more than fifty years.

She looked around the living room. It was chilly in

there, with no fire to warm it. I had never seen our living room without a fire blazing halfway up the chimney. Even in the height of the hottest summer my mother got up at the crack of dawn and lit the fire – not because she was cold but because a fire was necessary if there was to be hot water or an oven to cook their meals in.

'I expect he's outside feeding the pigs, or chopping sticks or something,' she said, looking closely into his worm-eaten wooden armchair. 'He was here not a minute ago bringing mud in on his boots, but where he is now I wouldn't like to say.' I stared at her, suddenly aware of what had happened. My mother had always ruled the roost with as firm a hand as my father would allow. Though he had never let her henpeck him, he gave in to her tempestuous ways until the way became too tempestuous for him to tolerate it any longer, then with a quick lift of the chin he would assert his position as head of the house. 'Tha can shut up now, Missis, tha's said plenty,' was all he needed to say to shut her up. She knew just how far she could go with him before he lifted his chin to her. But none of this had prepared me for the change that came over her once the head of the house had left it.

'The telegram said he was ill,' I told her, trying to bring her back to the reality she didn't want to face.

She laughed scornfully.

'Him ill?' she said. 'Your father's never been ill in his life, except for the time when that old cow up in the village nearly blinded him. Do you remember when she stuck her horn in his eye while he was milking her? Even then he wasn't what you could call ill. He didn't stop off work for weeks like the doctor told him he should. It would have taken more than an old cow like her to keep him away from work more than a day or two.' She looked again into his empty chair. 'It's a nuisance, he's never here when you want him. I'll give him a shout in a minute and tell him his dinner's ready.' There was no sign of dinner or any other meal being ready.

I realized that there was nothing to be gained by asking her more questions. Whatever had happened she was shutting her mind against admitting it. I got her hat and coat and we walked up the lane together to the farm where the farmer had squirted the children with new warm milk straight from the cow. It wasn't the same cow that had once nearly blinded my father.

The farmer and his wife told me that it was they who had sent the telegram, and that my father was in the County Hospital, too ill to be expected to live much longer. I went and sat beside his bed and waited until it was time to say goodbye to him. I didn't take my mother with me. The man who was lying in the bed would have been less real to her than the man who was outside somewhere feeding the pigs or chopping sticks.

She shouted often after that to remind him that his dinner was on the table, but she never seemed too surprised when he didn't come in for it. 'I'll put it in the oven and keep it hot for him,' she would say. Then she would wander aimlessly round the living room, not bothering to shout again for at least ten minutes.

I travelled a long way with my father to the place where they cremated him. My mother had always said that when their time came I was to have them cremated. I thought it was a terrible thing to do to a man who had always lived off the land. I would rather have left him lying peacefully somewhere beneath a tree than watch him disappear into the unknown through a curtain in the crematorium.

I sat and thought about him while the vicar, whom none of us knew, said kind things about a man he had never met. I remembered the way he had always called me Birdie, and the squeak of his leather leggings as we walked through the lanes and fields when I was a child. I thought of the day he had given me four half-crowns from the little leather bag he always carried in his trouser pocket, and how I had kissed his stubbly cheek before I climbed up on to the carrier's cart to leave home and go to be a nurse.

I couldn't tell what my mother was thinking, but it must have been very sad. The tears were pouring down her cheeks.

When it was time for me to go home to my family, I got up after a sleepless night. 'You'll have to leave here and come and live with us,' I said, putting into words the thoughts that had kept me awake.

My mother stopped poking the fire that she had gone back to lighting at the crack of dawn and looked at me. I saw from the look that whatever else she didn't want to face, she had already come to terms with the suggestion I had just made to her.

'I'll not come to live with you nor anybody else,' she said, giving the poker a rest for a moment. 'I shall stop where I am. This is my home and this is where I belong. Besides, what would your father say if I went gadding off and leaving him like that? He's never had to fend for himself, and he wouldn't know how to start.' She wielded the poker again and the subject was closed.

I left her there, with promises from the kind farmer's wife up the lane and some kind cousins up in the village that they would keep an eye on her for me, and that the moment they thought it was necessary for her to come and live with me, however much she resisted the idea, they would let me know. They also said they would see about getting her a dog to keep her company through the long winter nights and go for walks with her when she felt like walking. The dog might also protect her against unwelcome visitors, though not many visitors, welcome or unwelcome, trailed down the lane and up the cart-track unless there was some good purpose for the trail. And the shabbiness of the smallholding held out little promise for a burglar bent on getting rich quick.

It was longer than I had expected it to be before my mother came to live with us. She was a lady of spirit. She always had been. The letters I got from those who were keeping an eye on her for me told me that she had gone back to doing the things she had always done around the house, though the fender was never as burnished as it was while my father was alive.

The dog was a comfort to her, they said. She talked to it as if it were human. I spent a few uneasy moments thinking about that. Davies and I had once lodged with a very old lady who had a dog that she used to talk to as if it were human. She took the dog to bed with her every night and it snored beside her between the sheets. I didn't like to ask my mother's visitors if she did the same. If she did, I felt I would rather not know about it, and if she didn't, they would think me crazy for asking. They may not have known that lonely old ladies sometimes did things like that, if they were lonely enough and loved their dog and needed something warm to fill the empty space in their lives and in the double bed that was far too big for one.

I had a lot to do when I got home. I had already written to the Matron telling her about the telegram and extending my leave by a week. I spent the extra time cooking things for the family to eat so that there wouldn't be too much for me to cook when I came home too tired to throw the ingredients together and I went round the house with dusters and polishing rags, determined to go on night duty leaving floors that were clean enough to eat off, however far they had fallen below the standard by the time I came off duty again. I, who had always been so far behind with the house-work, suddenly caught up with it to a degree that astonished the family.

I also spent the last few minutes while I was tucking the children up at bedtime telling them that I was going to be a night nurse instead of a day nurse and warning them that they must be good girls for Daddy and not call too often for drinks, or wake screaming from a bad dream, or do anything that would ruin his chances of getting through the following day without falling asleep at his desk. I reminded them that daddies were different from mummies. Mummies had more stamina. They were the stronger sex.

The nearer night duty came, the more nervous I began to get about it. I started thinking about all the night duties I had done in the past, when there were more than forty patients in each of the long wards and I the only nurse on one of them. I thought of the man who had jumped to his death while I was too caught up with the other patients to know that he had even left his bed. I remembered a night sister at my training school who had crept round the wards in plimsolls hoping to catch one of her nurses nodding. And after I had thought of all these things I felt less and less like going on night duty.

But I cheered up a lot after I remembered the nights when Brown and I had worked together up at the Sanatorium. They were happy nights. We had shared the work and the responsibilities, the disasters and the lighter side, and had gone off duty in the morning too tired to eat our breakfast, but not too tired to laugh about the dirty story one of the men had told us while we were sponging him down in the middle of the night, or about the awful clatter that had sent us rushing to the entrance door only to discover that the noise was two hedgehogs making mad passionate love. If the nights at the fever hospital were anything like those nights they might not be too bad after all. I threw myself into preparing for them with renewed vigour.

On the first evening that I was to get on my bicycle and pedal away to work I listened attentively to the children's prayers – it was summertime and the midday sun had warmed the bedrooms – then I tucked them up, kissed them, gave them one or two further words of warning and went, leaving their father to shoulder the responsibility of looking after two sleeping children single-handed for the rest of the night. Until then there had been a defining line drawn between his duties as a father and mine as a mother. The line was rarely crossed. I washed for them, cooked for them, bathed them and listened to their prayers; he was the bread-winner, keeping them fed, clothed and still believing in Santa Claus. The bit of bread I brought in with the weekly pay packet hadn't done anything to confuse the two roles. But suddenly he was having to be mother as well as father. The strain of it was already telling on him when I turned the first corner. He gave me a feeble wave and walked back into the house; I could almost see the lines of care that were etched on his face.

The locker room was packed. There were nurses I knew and others I had never seen before. Another ward of geriatrics had been brought from the main hospital while I was away, and some of the nurses who came with them had also volunteered to go on night duty. They were the ones I knew. The staff from the fever side were strangers to me.

While I was putting on my white coat with the navy blue epaulettes I listened to the talk that was going on around me. None of it was very encouraging. It made me feel tired even before I had started work. Most of it was centred on the fact that the one who was talking hadn't had a wink of sleep all day. Something had always happened at the moment they were dropping off – the man had come to read the meter, the Jehovah's Witnesses had come to convert them and stayed for hours, or the neighbours were noisy and forgot there was a night nurse next door trying to get some sleep.

It occurred to me while I was listening that I hadn't had a wink of sleep either that day. Once, during the afternoon, I had sat down on a chair and put my feet up on another but the moment I shut my eyes the baker knocked at the door. I had always given the baker a cup of tea when he called, and it seemed churlish to turn him away just because I happened to be going to work that night. He didn't finish drinking the tea until it was time for me to fetch the children from school. Then it was time to do all the other things that had to be done.

'I haven't had a wink of sleep either today,' I said to the nurse who had the next locker to mine and was struggling into a coat with pale blue epaulettes. The struggle was putting a tremendous strain on the coat. It was a size sixteen, and she was a majestic twenty. She was built in a way which made lesser women feel fat: the flesh she had was arranged so neatly that none of it seemed in the least superfluous. There was a lot where a lot should be dwindling to proportionate amounts in other places. I envied her. I went in where I should have come out and had hills where there should have been plains.

She looked at me. The look was not a friendly one.

'But you didn't need any sleep today, did you?' she said frostily. 'You were in bed last night.' Overwhelmed with guilt that I had dared to compare my well-slept self with her night-starved weariness, I arranged the starkly plain cap on my head and went to report on duty.

Chapter Fourteen

DURING THE NEXT ten years that I spent as a part-time night nurse, wife and mother combined, I seemed almost to be living in two worlds. The moment I waved goodbye to the family in the evening and pedalled away to work I became a nurse. When I came off duty in the morning and pedalled home, I stopped at the paper shop to pay the paper bill, shouted good morning to the milkman and anybody else I met on the way that I happened to know, and was a housewife again, albeit a weary housewife. When I got into the house and scolded the children for throwing their nightdresses down on the floor instead of folding them tidily and putting them under their pillow as I had told them to the night before, I forgot that I was a nurse and became once more a mother. Only if the most terrible things had happened between the time I pedalled away and the time I pedalled home did I allow them to stay in my thoughts and merge the separate worlds into one.

The night duty I was doing was unlike any night duty I had ever done before. Because most of the nurses I worked with were wives and mothers as well, we had many things in common. We could sit over a cup of tea in the kitchen when there was nothing too pressing to be done and boast about our children's progress at school, gloss lightly over our husband's shortcomings and exchange tips on how to renovate an old suite to make it look like something out of the Ideal Home Exhibition without a penny being spent on it. (The penny had often already been spent on it by a naughty baby or a playful puppy.) Listening to the others tell of their domestic difficulties made our own so much easier to bear. When the sweet-faced assistant nurse who was a cross between the Mona Lisa and the Madonna fell over a bed laughing one night, I asked her what was so funny. The night had been hard, we were both tired and there seemed nothing much to laugh about.

'I threw a bowl of cornflakes at Henry this morning,' she spluttered.

Henry was her husband. He looked almost as saintly as she did. It was hard to imagine a battle of cornflakes being fought out between them. But I was glad she had told me about it. I had thrown a cup of tea at my husband the morning before and was racked with remorse. The remorse was made worse by the fact that the cup had missed him and hit the newly papered dining room wall instead. It had cost a lot of money to have the dining room papered, it would cost a lot more to have it papered again. The damage caused by the teacup had spread and there wasn't a scrap of the new wallpaper left to replace the bespattered lengths.

The night sister who came on the ward and asked us why we were laughing added to the fun by telling us of the time when her husband had papered their dining room. On the very same day one of their children had tripped and fallen with a plateful of liver and bacon and sent the whole lot streaming down the flocked wall. The tragedies when they happened might have been earth-shaking but they became far less so after they had been laughed over in the night.

Most of us part-timers were honest enough to admit that the only reason we were coming out to work was because there was never enough money to pay the bills. Those who said otherwise were looked at with suspicion, or branded at once as liars. When a new staff nurse reported on duty one night and told us that she was only there for the experience, we looked at her laddered stockings and shabby shoes and thought otherwise. We were glad when she finally owned up and admitted that she had come back to work to help pay off the mortgage.

Another nurse told us, with her nose in the air, that the money she earned wasn't really needed at home but would go towards paying for the parquet floors they were having laid in the mansion-type house she assured us she lived in.

'What are parky floors?' whispered Lynch to me. She was the auxiliary who was on duty that night with the rich new nurse and me.

'It's just a posh name for wood blocks,' I told her, not too sure myself what they were. We had Axminster at home, and not even wall to wall.

The nurse who came to work to subsidize the flooring was quick to point out that wood blocks were to parquet as rabbit was to mink. Soon she stopped talking about her floors and began to boast about the ballgown her husband had promised to buy her for ladies' night at the Masonic.

'What's the Masonic?' whispered Lynch.

'It's something terribly secret and you're not supposed to talk about it,' I told her, remembering an uncle-in-law who had allegiances to the Brotherhood but would never talk about it, however much we pestered him for details.

'Then why is she talking about it?' asked Lynch. I wasn't sure. It would have been uncharitable to say that the reason she talked so much about her different lifestyle was in order to impress us with it. We tried not to be too impressed but when she went into great detail about the hundred-guinea operation she had just had, we who had

had the same operation under the National Health really began to feel like paupers. It was a relief to us all when she borrowed a pound off one of us to see her through the end of the week and we realized that she had come back to work for the money exactly like the rest of us.

Because the fever hospital was small, there were no domestics on duty at night and nobody to cook or serve our meals. Large trays of food were sent across to the wards in the daytime ready for the night staff to do their worst with at midnight. Any cooking that had to be done was usually done by whichever nurse on each ward could best be trusted to fry a sausage or boil a potato in the kitchen at the same time as she was doing something terribly important for a patient in the ward. The banana custard or stale cake trifle that we usually got for pudding didn't have to be cooked so could come to no harm, even if something awful happened when we were in the middle of eating it.

Something awful quite often happened to ruin our midnight meal. Even if nothing awful happened, the meal was frequently interrupted by an urgent call from a patient that turned out not to be urgent after all, or by a loud bang which would make us jump from the table in panic and rush into the ward expecting to find somebody on the floor. For a patient to fall out of bed while we were eating in the kitchen would have been shocking enough to keep us guiltily awake the next day and perhaps for many days after that, despite the fact that it was perfectly legal to eat our midnight meal in the kitchen. But fortunately very few people ever fell out of bed and there was usually a simple explanation for the bang we had heard: a dropped beaker full of teeth, or the entire contents of a locker crashing to the floor after a failed attempt at reaching for a biscuit. But discovering that the thud was falling teeth and not a falling patient didn't stop us from leaping from the table when we heard another thud. That none of us got ulcers could only have been because nurses are used to gulping down their food. They have done it for so long, to give them a chance to do other things, that eating at leisure seems a waste of time. Their stomachs have become adjusted over the years to being abused.

It was a week or two before I could sit and eat a two-course meal in the kitchen without expecting a hand to fall on my shoulder and a stern voice telling me to report to the Matron in the morning for my sins. The first night I was back at work I asked anxiously what would happen if the night sister came and caught us eating corned beef and beetroot in the kitchen. (Nobody had volunteered to cook the potatoes so we were having to live without them.)

The night sister answered the question herself by walking into the kitchen just as I asked it. When I sprang up from my chair, ashamed at being caught sitting in it, she mistook the reflex action for kindness and threw herself down on the vacant seat. I saw then that she was one of us. Though she wore a night sister's uniform she looked too motherly not to be a mother and too tired to have had more than a wink of sleep all day – if indeed she had even had that. The size twenty nurse who had followed me on to the ward when I reported on duty offered her a cup of tea, which she accepted as gratefully as the chair I wasn't exactly offering her.

She refused the bowl of stale-cake trifle we tried to tempt her with – she was on a diet that night, she said. I was also on a diet that night, and so was the size twenty nurse. We sat for a while discussing the merits of the various diets we had tried. We had tried them all. We bought packets of slimming biscuits and ate the lot at one sitting; we drank bottlesful of a special sort of vinegar that we foolishly believed would melt our too-solid flesh away like wax from a burning candle; we went on the grapefruit diet, the banana diet and the boiled egg diet. The boiled egg diet was the worst one of them all. We ate so many hard boiled eggs while we were on the diet that our breath started to smell like the sulphuric gases from a spouting geyser. We also became very constipated.

None of the diets ever worked for me. They might perhaps have been more successful if I hadn't followed each day's dieting with an orgy of eating that more than made up for the deprivations I suffered while I was on the diet.

After the night sister had drunk her tea and put her shoes back on again we went round the ward. As we walked slowly from bed to bed I realized again the vast difference there was between being a full-time and resident nurse and coming back to hospital part-time, married and a mother to boot. I had learned while I was on day duty up at the main hospital that if the old lady who lived at the end of the road were we lived was suddenly admitted to a bed on the ward where we worked, she was still the old lady from the end of our road. If she was the kind old lady who gave the children a smile and a liquorice all-sort when they walked past her house on their way to school, we rewarded her for her kindness by seeing that she got a warm bedpan whenever she asked us for a bedpan, and a needle without a fish hook on the end of it when we gave her an injection. But if she was the crabby old thing who waved a threatening stick at every child who passed her gate, we issued warning notices about her to whoever else would be having to nurse her. 'I should watch out for her if I were you. She lives down our road and she's a bit of a tartar.' And though the warnings were heeded, the old lady still got warm bedpans and needles with no fish hooks on the end. We had met people like her before. We knew that anybody who waved her stick at children would wave the big stick at us for even the slightest neglect or the most imagined slight. We were careful to see that she wasn't neglected or slighted in any way at all.

The sister stopped at one of the beds. The patient in it was lying quite still with her eyes wide open.

'Hello, Emma,' the sister said, sounding almost as if she were greeting somebody over her garden wall. 'Why aren't you asleep? It's long past your bedtime isn't it?' Emma smiled with her eyes but her mouth didn't move. The sister chatted to her for a few minutes about her family, then moved on.

'Her family lives near me,' she said, when we were safely past the bed. 'It's all very sad, really. She hates being in here but her daughter's been looking after her at home since she had the stroke two years ago. Even with the district nurse going in twice a day it was more than she could cope with, with a husband and two children as well. It's all right people talking about sons and daughters having a duty to care for their parents when they get old, but it isn't always easy having somebody lying in a bed in the sitting room for years. It can often break up a home.'

While the sister was talking, I thought of my own mother and wondered how I would manage when I got the letter telling me that she would have to come and live with us however much she rebelled against the idea. I knew that if things were bad enough for the letter to be sent, there was a possibility of our sitting room at home having to be turned into a single-bedded chronic ward overnight. There would be extra washing to do, the children would have to keep their friends quiet when they came visiting and nobody would be able to have a good row in case it upset my mother to hear raised voices. As in most households everybody in ours needed a good row sometimes to clear the air. It was better to have the row and get it over than to preserve an explosive silence. Things were going to be no easier for me than they were for Emma's daughter.

I realized also while I was thinking that it was a great help to a nurse in understanding her patient's problems if she had had some of the problems herself. The midwife with children of her own is less likely to tell the panting mother-to-be in the labour room that the pains she says she is feeling aren't really pains at all but little contractions that will go away if the pants are the right size. The mother who is also a nurse doesn't waste her breath advising a harassed mother to put her feet up for several hours a day when she gets home after her operation. The nurse knows from experience that when the mother gets home there will be piles of washing everywhere and masses of fingermarks on the paintwork.

A harassed mother once told me what happened to her when she went home from hospital after an operation that was serious enough to leave her weak at the knees but not serious enough to earn her the luxury of a week at a convalescent home. Very slowly she had gone round the house, taking in the piles of washing everywhere and noting the masses of fingerprints on the paintwork. When she got to the kitchen she had lifted up her eyes to the ceiling and seen with dismay the greasy grime that had collected there over a week or two of fry-ups that her family had lived on while she was away. Being as house-proud as Selina, she had averted her eyes from the ceiling until she could avert them no longer, and then got together a chair, a bucket of sudsy water and a wash rag. Halfway across the ceiling she came over faint, climbed off the chair and lay down on the floor looking up at the ceiling. The half she had washed stood out so sharply from the half she hadn't that when the faintness passed she got back on to the chair and finished the job.

When the family came in from school and home from the office they were overjoyed that she was back with them again. They fell upon the dinner she cooked for them, entreating her as they ate it to take things easy and put her feet up for several hours a day and not to bother about cooking meals for them; they would rather starve than have her ill again. None of them even noticed the ceiling, but they all asked for second help-ings of the pudding she had made.

I believed every word of it. I knew it was the sort of thing that happened to mothers when they went home after a spell in hospital. Being a part-time nurse gave me a better understanding of things like that.

'Where's Harriet?' I asked the sister, when we came to the bed that Harriet was put into after the move from the main hospital.

'She's back up there again,' said the sister. 'She broke her hip one day while she was hopping to the lavatory.'

I wasn't a bit surprised to hear it. Harriet had lost a leg in a car crash when she was seventy-nine. Somebody had suggested that she should have an artificial leg fitted, and though Harriet said she didn't want a wooden leg and wouldn't wear one even if they gave her one, nobody took any notice of her. She was seventy-nine and past the age of being able to make decisions for herself. She went to a limb-fitting centre where they gave her a shiny new leg that did most of the things her own leg had done before it was chopped off in the car crash. They showed her how to kick footballs about with it and how to walk through parallel bars with it strapped on to her stump. The day at last came when they told her she had passed whatever test they had set and she was now perfectly capable of living a normal life with the new bright shining leg. She lived a normal life with it for just as long as it took her to get up the ward in the main hospital where she was a patient, then she unstrapped all the strappings, put the leg behind her locker and never strapped it on again. She showed it to her visitors with the same look of pride on her face as she wore when she showed them the set of gleaming false teeth that she kept in her sponge bag. She had been just as firm with those who had suggested the teeth as she was with those who suggested the leg. She said quite clearly that she wouldn't lower herself by filling her mouth with such rubbish. The leg and the teeth were gifts from the National Health Service, and must have given more joy to the giver than they did to the one who received them. A lot of time and money might have been saved if Harriet had been listened to when she declared that she didn't want either of them, and she would still have broken her hip hopping to the lavatory, and suffered with chronic indigestion through not being able to chew her food properly.

I walked with the sister across the grounds and over to the fever side where she had her office. It was a dark night. Somewhere a long way off a dog barked, and somewhere in a tree nearby an owl hooted. The dimmed lights of the cubicle wards shone out feebly in the blackness and as we got to the door an ambulance drove quietly up and stopped.

'Another admission,' groaned the sister. 'That's the third one tonight. There's a lot of gastroenteritis about.' She went through the door and an ambulance man followed her, carrying a baby wrapped up in a red blanket. The father and mother got out of the ambulance, and I saw that the mother was crying. I went back to my own ward, glad that the admission wasn't for us.

The one thing that the night duty I was doing now had in common with all the other night duty I had ever done was that we didn't get any official time off. We were on from eight in the evening until eight in the morning and whatever rest we had depended entirely on how many nurses were on duty and how busy the ward was. If nothing catastrophic was happening, we divided the time between our midnight meal and the first rush of the morning work and took it in turns to go into the ward office, unfasten our belts, take off our shoes and sit down on the very uncomfortable office chair.

I only once went into the office for a rest and the rest was a very short one. The windows in the office were large and uncurtained. In the daytime they looked out on to acres of fields that had once been a flourishing market garden, but since the market garden had fallen on hard times, there were now only acres of weeds and tall grasses. In the night the windows looked out on to nothing but blackness. Because they were on ground level it was easy for a vivid imagination to fill the blanks of the glass panes with leering faces and staring eyes. I had a vivid imagination. Though I never actually saw the leering faces and staring eyes, I knew they were there. When the office clock suddenly stopped ticking I looked for the hand that had stopped it and waited for one of the leering faces to leer out at me. Then I grabbed my belt, picked up my shoes and fled back to the kitchen.

'You can have my rest period as well as your own,' I said to Lynch and the rich staff nurse. 'I'll sit here in the kitchen.'

But even the kitchen had its terrors for me. The acres of weeds and tall grasses were the haunt of millions of great white moths. When they saw the light shining from the kitchen window they came across and beat against the glass, imploring me to let them in so that they could singe their wings at the light. The fury of the beating wings and the writhing mass of moths filled me with a superstitious terror that was as bad as the terror of the unseen faces at the office windows. I had read somewhere that in every seagull lies the soul of a sailor drowned at sea. I knew beyond doubt that in each of the moths there was a soul pleading to come into the kitchen. I also knew that across the road from the overgrown fields was the cemetery into which Lynch and other passengers had led the bus driver when the smog was on. There were plenty of souls in there to keep the moths flapping their wings for a long time.

None of the other nurses seemed to mind the moths, nor were they driven from the office by staring eyes and unseen faces, but all of them except Brown had their own small fears. Brown was far too sensible to fear things that weren't there or to see more than was apparent on the surface. But the size twenty nurse, who looked as if she would eat little men for breakfast, trembled at the thought of being confronted by even a very little man whenever she had to walk across the isolation block to borrow something or to deliver a message to the night sister that couldn't be telephoned. And Lynch spent a lot of the night prowling round the ward looking for night prowlers.

The rich staff nurse was more nervous than any of us. 'God,' she would say, starting up from the table when we were eating our meal, 'I heard somebody knocking – it's a tramp trying to get in.' She would shiver and shake until one of us would go and unbolt the outer door to convince her that there was no tramp trying to get in. But five minutes later she would start up again. 'There's somebody creeping along the corridor – I can hear him breathing.' Again one of us would have to go out and come back with the news that the only thing stirring in the corridor was a field mouse that had come in when we opened the door to see if there was a tramp on the step.

But with all the rich staff nurse's fears of tramps and masculine heavy breathing, and Lynch's night prowlers (which she always assumed were men) and all the other strange men who were waiting to pounce on the size twenty nurse, it wasn't a man who came in terror to our door one night. It was a young girl, who had once been pretty.

Brown was the first to hear the hammering on the door. We were busy in the ward. There would be no rest for any of us that night. Mrs Love was dying, and a patient who had been admitted during the day was having to have a constant watch kept over her to stop her from pulling out tubes that were vital to her recovery. She clawed at the connection that was dripping fluid into her arm and tried to push away the oxygen without which she would have joined Mrs Love in her dying. We were having a hard job persuading her that she had still a lot to live for. She certainly hadn't thought so when she shut all her doors and windows at home and turned on the gas taps – unless, of course, it was a cry for help, which it might have been since she turned on the taps only a few minutes before the district nurse was due to come to give her her weekly bath. The district nurse said she wasn't a bit surprised to find the gas taps on. The old lady had fretted ever since her only son went off to America. She knew it would be the last she ever saw of him, so there was nothing left worth living for. But she lived for a long time after that, and was quite happy to sit on a chair in the ward watching what was going on around her. She even found strength to argue with old Mrs Sweetman one day, but she lost the argument.

After Brown had drawn my attention to the hammering on the ward door we both went and opened it. The young girl who fell at our feet had been severely beaten up. Until that night she had foolishly thought that rape was something that only happened to girls in the Sunday papers. She had been walking alone along the lane when suddenly she was alone no longer. Her poor torn face told us of the struggle she put up to keep her innocence. The face would be scarred for life, but so would her mind. Rape wasn't something that only happened to girls in the Sunday papers; it was something that happened to girls who walked alone down the lane past the fever hospital on their way from the pictures after missing the last bus.

Winter came and the moths went away to do whatever moths do in the wintertime, and then one night the phone rang just as we were sitting down for our midnight meal. The staff nurse on one of the cubicle wards had put her foot through the chair she stood on to change a light bulb. She had done so much damage to her leg that she would need to be taken to the main hospital at once. I was to go across and take her place. I put the phone down slowly, and then I wrapped my cloak around me and went to report to the night sister on the isolation block.

Chapter Fifteen

Almost all nurses somewhere along their career have developed an immunity against catching things off their patients or have deluded themselves into thinking they have such a miraculous immunity. However often they are thrown into a hotbed of infection they still believe that they are not as other people and will rise from the hotbed unharmed. But in the early days of their training they are as afraid of catching things as any ordinary mortals. Davies and the Irish girl who did their training with me were quite nervous when it was their turn to face the dangers of VD or the risks of TB.

'Will I catch it?' Davies had asked anxiously while we were walking out to the Styx of the Sanatorium block. After I had assured her that there was every likelihood of her ending her days spitting up blood in an icy garret like Mimi, she at once started making plans for ending them instead in an expensive chalet high on a mountainside. She didn't fancy a garret, she said; she would prefer the more rarefied atmosphere of the Swiss Alps. Neither of us gave a thought to where she was going to find the money for such a luxurious death. Like me, she never had enough money to live on, never mind having to amass a fortune to ease her passage into the next world.

But we all knew that nothing so glamorous would result from a moment of carelessness while we were working on the VD wards. The Irish girl remembered pictures she had seen in medical books of advanced cases of syphilis. The thought of not having a nose on her twenty-first birthday terrified her.

Davies didn't go down with galloping consumption, and the worse thing that happened to the Irish girl's nose was the cold sore she got every winter. Soon their fears of catching things died down and they knew they had developed the miraculous immunity that is the birthright of every nurse.

I also had boasted that being a nurse protected me from assault by enemy infections. Nevertheless, I walked across to the fever side of the hospital with some reluctance. Though the Matron had warned us that we might be asked to go across there if an emergency arose, I had heard enough in the locker room to put me off the idea. It seemed there were still enough infectious diseases about to fill the cubicles and keep the nurses who worked in them busy – far too busy sometimes. I knew that the night life which lay ahead of me would be different altogether from the night life I was leaving behind on the female chronic ward. There were also thoughts of my family to trouble me. I had little nagging fears that I might not do all I should do to keep the infections confined to the cubicles, but would take one home with me to spread it around amongst my nearest and dearest. Then I reminded myself that I was a State Registered nurse and knew all the rules about nursing infectious diseases. If I kept to them strictly my family would come to no harm through me. I quickened my step and hurried through the dark grounds.

The sister – who was a wife and mother as well, and went on as many unsuccessful slimming diets as I did – took me into her office and gave me a quick run-through of the patients listed in the report book. Not all of them were children. Because each of the cubicles was an entirely separate small ward divided from the next by a discreetly curtained window, the patients in them could be of any age and either sex. These who were in that night were a typical assortment of the infectious diseases that were being brought in then to the fever hospital. Later the assortment became less typical, when different and more frightening things started coming in.

I listened carefully to the night sister's report on each patient, but it wasn't until we woke them up at five o'clock to take their temperatures, give them their antibiotics, bowls and bedpans, and ask them what they wanted for breakfast that I was able to get to know all of them properly, though long before five o'clock I felt I knew the three tiny babies who were in with gastroenteritis very well indeed. It had been a long time since I changed so many nappies and applied so much soothing cream to little red bottoms. I even had to be shown by the auxiliary nurse how to fold the nappies in the modern way, how to mix the feeds and how to persuade the babies that the weak dilution we were offering them was as much to their taste as the rich full-flavoured milk they had been accustomed to getting. None of the babies we had in that night was seriously ill, but they were ill enough to cause me a little maternal anxiety as well as a nurse's concern. Thinking of my own children at home, hopefully sleeping and dreaming of nice things, made the restless babies in their cots rather more than mere patients, if a little less than my own children. It was yet another of the changed attitudes to nursing that I found even more marked on the fever side, where we were often wives and mothers as well as nurses.

In the cubicle next to the kitchen there was a young man, yellow with an acutely infectious liver complaint, who went black with anger at being offered only a slice of dry toast and a cup of milkless tea for his breakfast.

When he asked why he couldn't have egg and bacon like the other patients who were getting it as a special treat because it was Sunday, we did our best to explain that the fatty bacon and fried egg would do terrible things to his liver. He made such a fuss that Sister suggested we should fill a plate with the fattiest bacon we could find and take it in to him. He turned a deeper shade of yellow at the sight of it and believed us then that a slice of dry toast would do him a lot more good. But later, when we were in another cubicle, we talked about the man with the liver and said how sorry we were for him. It must be awful, we said, to only have a slice of dry toast for your breakfast when you were hungry enough to eat a horse. We forgave him for the fuss he had made. All of us except the very senior assistant nurse had men of our own at home. We knew what a fuss they made if they didn't get what they wanted. The man with the liver hadn't had what he wanted for a long time – he had every right to make a fuss.

Next to the man with the liver, a boy of fifteen lay in bed, sick at the thought of having to lie in bed when he should have been at home swotting for his mock GCE. The high fever and tender swollen glands that had brought him into the isolation hospital seemed a poor excuse for having to stay there when he so desperately needed to astonish his teachers with his amazing grasp of the facts they had been drumming into him over the years. Again the mothers among us were able to understand and sympathize.

'It's a pity he had to get glandular fever when he should have been swotting for his exams,' said the less-senior assistant nurse, who had boys of her own that were swotting for their exams. 'It'll put him back a lot when he goes back to school next term.' The nurse saw the illness as a debilitating disease; the mother saw it as a hindrance to the boy's academic achievements. It would have been hard to tell which of the two she thought would do him most harm. The kind senior assistant nurse had no doubts at all. 'You forget about exams and things and just think about getting better,' she told him, giving him some science fiction to read and taking away the history book his mother had brought in for him. His mother was very concerned that he wouldn't be better in time to sit his exams. She kept bringing in school books, forgetting they would have to stay in there, since it was an isolation hospital she was bringing them to.

They told me that the old soldier in cubicle ten, who kept ringing his bell, had been admitted many times. Because everybody liked him nobody minded him ringing his bell so often. He shivered his nights away with recurring attacks of the malaria that had plagued him since he was bitten by a mosquito in a steamy jungle a long way from home. The memories of the jungle came back to him vividly while he was trying to stop shaking. He needed a lot of reassuring before he would let whoever had answered his last bell leave him to go and answer another. He had stopped being a soldier a long time ago and was just a pitiful old man.

Along the corridor and next to the medical room was a woman with shingles. Three cubicles away from her there was another woman with shingles. They were both very relieved that the shingles hadn't encircled their waists and met somewhere in the middle. Like my mother they had a deeply rooted superstition about shingles. They knew that if the ends of the circle became entwined nothing could save them: they were doomed to die. One of the ladies had an eye so severely damaged by the shingles that it had to be removed, but she still clung to the old superstition. 'Never mind,' she said, when they told her about the eye. 'It could have been worse. If the shingles had met round my waist I'd be dead.' The belief was to sustain her through years of semi-blindness.

The little boy who lay in the cubicle opposite the office had been lying there for a long time. He was admitted when he was only four with one of the simple infectious diseases that children didn't die of any more, and which didn't usually have to be nursed in a fever hospital. He died when he was seven, still in the coma he was in the night he was admitted. For three years he had been cared for devotedly by everybody who came and went on the ward, but most devotedly by one of the assistant nurses on day duty. She gave him all the love she would have given to a child of her own if she had ever been married and had a child. It made no difference to her that he was in a coma and never responded to the love.

'But why wasn't he sent home?' I asked. 'Why did the doctor keep him here?'

I should have known the answer before I asked the question. The fever side of the hospital had no allegiances to the main hospital, despite the fact that the staff was interchangeable. The geriatrics were still under the care of the doctors who had always visited them; the fever side had as its medical officer: a very large, very kind and very Jewish doctor. He was the rock upon which we all leaned whenever we needed a rock to lean on. He never let us down. He never let the patients down either. When he saw that the little boy in the cubicle opposite the office would be better there than in a bigger, more impersonal place, he talked to the poor young mother and promised her that her son would have all the care he needed for as long as he needed it, and he kept his promise. When the little boy died, the doctor turned his head away so that none of us would see his tears.

Each of the cubicles was a small and separate world with its own small and separate histories. Many of the histories stayed in the memory for one reason or another. We remembered the youth who was admitted to cubicle two one night because he was a burglar by trade, and by some strange coincidence, one of the non-resident nurses had been burgled for the second time just before he was admitted. She was also the nurse who came on duty an hour too early one autumn morning because she had forgotten to put her clocks back as the wireless and the newspapers told her to. She started forgetting to do a lot of things after she had been burgled for the second time. Being burgled once is bad enough, but for a burglar to take two bites of the same cherry can change a healthy nervous system into a bundle of neuroses overnight. She found it hard to stay professionally detached whenever she did anything to the patient in cubicle two. 'I feel like using a blunt needle every time I give him his penicillin,' she confessed to us when she was giving us the report one evening. 'I know it wasn't him who burgled me, but I feel like making him pay for whoever did.'

I tried to find out from him why he and others like him did things that caused other people so much unhappiness.

'Why do you do it,' I asked, then waited, foolishly expecting an answer.

'Just for a giggle,' he said, sounding surprised that I didn't know.

'But don't you ever think of the people you rob and the pain it causes them, especially if they can't afford to be robbed?' The nurse who had been burgled couldn't afford to be robbed. The things she was robbed of were treasures that were only precious to her for the pleasure they gave her, but that made them very valuable.

'That's their look out, innit?' he said. 'I don't bother about things like that.' He paused for a moment, and then gave me a pleading look. 'Is there anything to eat in the kitchen? The supper was rotten tonight, and I'm starving.' I went to the kitchen and found him some bread and cheese. He was a growing boy as well as a burglar, and I knew the supper had been rotten – we were having the remains of it for our midnight meal.

I never found out why burglars burgled people, unless they did it for a bit of a giggle, but there had to be more in it for some of them than just a giggle.

The two young car thieves who were admitted from the same remand home as the boy burglar, and with the same very minor infection, were no more helpful when I tried to get at the root of what made them steal cars. If people were daft enough to leave their cars unlocked, then they could expect to have them pinched, they said.

'But you pinch cars that haven't been left unlocked,' I said, thinking of a neighbour who treated his car like a baby, bathing it every Saturday and polishing off each tiny speck as it appeared. He was a broken man when it disappeared from outside his house one Saturday evening only an hour after he had bathed it. He never got it back, which was just as well. The things that car thieves sometimes do to the cars they steal would have put the poor man in his grave if they had done them to his car.

'Would you steal the doctor's car if you saw him leave it in the street unlocked one day?' I asked them, knowing that they liked the ward doctor as much as I did, as much as everybody on the fever side did.

'No, we wouldn't steal his car,' one of them said, looking and sounding disgusted with me for suggesting something so outrageous. 'We only nick little cars that can't be recognized easy. He's got a bloody great Jag.'

I was very disappointed. From the look of disgust and the tone of voice I had assumed that the reason they wouldn't dream of stealing the doctor's car was because he was kind and good and treated them with the same respect he gave to all his patients, whether they were burglars, car thieves or just plain ordinary people.

The two car thieves ran away one evening. I saw them streaking out of the side entrance to the hospital when I was biking through the main entrance on my way to the locker room. It took me a moment to realize what was happening and another moment to get round to the other gate, and by then they were nowhere in sight. The day sister was not amused when I burst into her office to tell her that two of her patients were her patients no longer. It had been a long and tiring day for her. There were a lot of small infectious diseases going about, the Emergency Bed Service had been ringing up all day demanding emergency beds, and she was suffering from menopausal depression aggravated by worry. It wasn't a good time to tell her that two of her beds were now empty and would be available for the Emergency Bed Service the next time they rang.

The remand home from where the boys were admitted were very cross with us for letting them get away, but the day sister had a sharp tongue when she was roused and she was easily roused. She reminded the remand home that we were a hospital and not a prison, and if they didn't let their inmates catch infectious diseases the situation would never have arisen anyway, and then she slammed the phone down and vented her menopausal anger on me. Luckily the infection the boys had was no longer infectious, but one or two cars disappeared from outside one or two houses before the police managed to round up those who had stolen them.

When Charlie was brought in too drunk to know that he was being brought in, the ambulance men told us that a doctor at the police station thought he had a skin disease that might be catching. We all knew Charlie. He was usually to be seen reeling around the town brandishing a bottle and picking a fight with anybody willing to fight with him. He disrupted bus queues, did naughty things behind bushes in the park and was exceedingly kind to old ladies who looked as if they wanted to get across the road. He could hold up a stream of traffic for several minutes while he staggered in front of it with the old lady in tow. When he reached the other side he would bow deeply, kiss her hand in the most courteous way imaginable and leave her, and then make rude gestures to the angry drivers who had to wait while he performed his 'being kind to old ladies' act. It turned out that he did have a skin disease that was catching. He was in with us for quite a while. He was a good patient, courteous and intelligent. Lynch went into his cubicle one night when she had been sent over to relieve our usual auxiliary. She looked at him in wonder.

'And is it sober you are for a change?' she said. He gave her a small, hurt smile. He was very sensitive about his drunkenness when he was sober. 'God knows why you always have to be drunk when you're not a bad sort of chap at all without the drink in you.'

He thought about what she had said for a moment, and then he gave her his explanation for the state he was usually in when we saw him in the town. 'Lady,' he said solemnly, 'some men love God, and some love women. I drink.' He drank the warm milk we gave him, and then we turned out his light and left him. We had just closed the cubicle door when we heard him call. Lynch opened the door again. 'Lady,' said Charlie, 'I don't suppose either of you would care to kiss me goodnight?'

Lynch shut the door with a bang, and then fell about on the corridor laughing. 'He's got no drink so he's started to love women instead!' she choked.

I saw him once or twice in the town after he was discharged. Then I saw him no more but I read about him in the local paper. He had picked a fight with a bigger man than himself and was already dead when they got him into the accident and emergency department at the main hospital. The manslaughter charge didn't stick. Charlie would have died even if he hadn't been knocked down. His brain was so softened by drink, or his arteries were so hardened by it, that he was lucky to have lived so long. Thinking about him while I was reading the local paper, and remembering what a good patient he was and how nice he could be when he was sober, made me wish he had stayed sober and alive after he left the fever hospital. Lynch said maybe she should have given the poor old devil a kiss after all, but I told her not to feel guilty about it; after all, she was a married woman as well as a nurse, and he had got a contagious skin infection.

I spent the rest of my work session, after Charlie went out, 'specialling' Katherine. 'Specialling' meant having to stay in her cubicle from the moment I went on duty to the moment I came off, doing nothing else but the things that had to be done for her. Katherine was a child with Down's syndrome. She was nine. She came in bloated and jaundiced with a virus disease she had caught while she was paddling in the stream near her home. The stream was the swimming pool for all the local rats. It was they who had bestowed the virus disease upon Katherine.

For a while it seemed that Katherine wouldn't be strong enough to fight off the infection and her parents came in each evening to sit with her until I sent them home saying that we would let them know if there was any change in her condition before they rang up in the morning. When they took off their masks and gowns and went home I almost regretted that I was a wife and mother as well as a nurse. I knew exactly how I would be feeling if the antibiotics that could work miracles weren't working any miracles on my child. At the end of the night I biked home almost too tired to see the way, and too tired to do more than nod when the family asked me whether I'd had a good night. Brightening the breakfast table with an account of the funny thing that had happened to a granny on her way to the lavatory wasn't the same as trying to tell them about the little girl who might not be there when I went back to work.

When Katherine started to get better, I understood

why children with Down's syndrome are so dearly loved by their parents.

'She wasn't born on the Sabbath day by any chance, was she?' I asked her mother, who wept with joy whenever she came into the cubicle and saw how much better Katherine looked.

'Yes, as a matter of fact she was,' she said. 'But how did you know?' I didn't know. All I knew was that Katherine was 'loving and kind and good and gay', as the little nursery rhyme says all children that were born on the Sabbath day turn out to be.

Her mother told me of the weary hours they had spent when Katherine was a baby, trying to make her take her feeds, and the even more weary hours they had spent as she got older teaching her the little things that come naturally to the children that people call 'normal'. Katherine gave us a beaming smile and I was glad she hadn't let the virus infection undo all the good work her parents had done.

While I was setting up the drips and doing all the other things that had to be done for her, I thought of my own children who sometimes took jam jars and fished for sticklebacks in the stream near Katherine's home. I never allowed them to do it again, and whenever I saw other children splashing barefoot in the murky water I called out warning things about the rats, but they never took any notice of me. They went on dabbling their feet in the stream, thinking I was just another interfering old busybody. They didn't realize that I was a part-time nurse who, because I was a mother as well, related things that I saw inside the hospital to things I saw happening outside.

There were other ways in which being a part-time nurse affected our lives outside the hospital. Resident nurses speed their departing patients with good wishes and a sincere hope, expressed in the friendliest terms, that they will never see them again. Non-resident nurses, and especially those who live in the town and go round the shops looking for bargains, are often stopped in the street by people they have once nursed who got better in spite of the nursing, or, more sadly, by the relatives of those who didn't get better. They are also given progress reports on past patients. Not all the reports give credit to the nursing. I was made to feel very guilty once by a woman who stopped me in the street. I hadn't seen her for a long time and didn't like her very much.

'Hello,' she said. 'You're down at the fever hospital, aren't you?'

I confessed that I was, and then waited for the adverse comments I had learned to expect from her.

'Do you remember that man you had in there a little while ago with something wrong with him?'

We had had a lot of men in there with something

wrong with them, some of them memorable, some of them not.

'Which man?' I asked. It took her a long time to separate the particular man from all the others, but suddenly I remembered him.

'Well,' she said, accusingly, 'he's never been the same since he was in there. He's started frightening girls on the towpath. He never used to do things like that. Not before he was down at the fever hospital.' And for some irrational reason I felt responsible for all the times our ex-patient had frightened girls on the towpath. It was as if my nursing had something to do with his little weakness. It would have been professionally unethical to tell her that he had his little weakness before ever he went into the fever hospital. He had admitted it to the night sister when she went into his cubicle one evening and he tried unsuccessfully to frighten her. She had been looking at the things he was showing her for too many years to be frightened by his little demonstration. But I could well see how the girls on the towpath might react. I escaped from the woman, feeling slightly bruised by the encounter, and wishing that our outside contact with our inside job didn't involve part-timers in such embarrassing encounters in the High Street or in the grocery store.

Nevertheless, there were times when we were allowed to forget we were nurses: times when we were

needed just because somebody needed a friend to turn
to and not a nurse to give them advice or to bear the
brunt of unfortunate happenings on the towpath. Such
a time came for me when a neighbour knocked at my
door early one morning and told me that her son was
dead. He had gone to bed a healthy young man and, for
a reason which his mother never quite understood, he
had stopped breathing sometime during the night. The
only comfort I could give her was the comfort from the
part of me that was a mother. I looked at the young
man lying so peacefully dead and thought of him as I
had seen him the day before: tall and strong, and with
good looks and a vintage car that made the young girls
sigh with longing and turned the old men green with
envy. Seeing him through a mother's eyes made his
death harder to bear than if I had only observed him
with the more professional detachment of a nurse on a
hospital ward. The nurse would have been filled with
pity, but I felt a little of the heartbreak that the young
man's mother was feeling.

We went on starving the patients who came in with
infective liver complaints, pumping antibiotics into
those who came in with things that would have killed
them before the days of antibiotics, and grieving over
babies who sometimes died however many antibiotics
we gave them. Those that didn't die went home ruined
by all the attention they had got from us during the

night. It was nice having a baby to cuddle after our own children had grown too old to want cuddling, and before they were old enough to give us grandchildren to cuddle. The babies in the cubicles filled the gap very satisfactorily.

Then suddenly, or maybe not so suddenly, a change started to come over the little wards on the fever side of the hospital, and a little colour started to come into our lives. New worlds were opened up. The colour and the new worlds were as strange to us at first as we were to the people who brought them. It took time for us all to adjust.

Part Five

Chapter Sixteen

I HAD BEEN working on the fever side for quite some time when the immigrants started landing in the country in numbers. The hospital was only a mile or two away from one of the major airports and soon there were almost as many immigrant patients being admitted to our cubicles as home-based ones. Some came in to us straight from the airport with a suspected infectious disease, an already confirmed infection, or because they were only vaccinated when they arrived in the country and would have to stay with us until their period of quarantine was over. Others came in from a nearby town which, because of its special needs and the nature of its industry, had become the promised land for a seemingly unending flow of Sikhs, Hindus and Muslims.

Turbans and saris gave the streets a bright new look and the lilt of Asian voices made a soft backing to the usual chorus of local vernacular; curry-scented air reached for the skies, and chapatis and poppadums were as much in demand as bread. Posters outside the cinemas that advertised Hollywood attractions were torn down and others put up in their place depicting exotic Asian ladies being wooed at a respectful distance by exotic Asian gentlemen. Shops closed down one week and opened up again the next under entirely new management. The new management was almost certain to be a smiling turbaned gentleman with his shy little wife, a child or two and a few close relatives peeping out of the small room at the back of the shop. The rooms they peeped from were as intriguing to us as we, with our pale skins and mousy hair, were to the peepers.

'You all look alike to me,' giggled an Asian patient one night after she had yet again confused two of the nurses who couldn't have looked less alike. Her remark surprised us. We had always thought that it was they who always looked alike.

As well as illness, the immigrants brought certain problems into our cubicles. The problems were mainly caused by religious and language differences, and were as difficult for the nurse to solve as they were for the patients. There were things that had to be accepted on both sides, and lessons to be learnt before any sort of trust was established between pale-faced nurse and darker-skinned patient. A lot of mistakes were made before the lessons were learned. When the not-so-senior assistant nurse was sent by a staff nurse to take the Hindu in cubicle two his medicine, she went back to the staff nurse with a puzzled look on her face.

'He's saying his prayers,' she said anxiously. 'He wouldn't look up when I went in. I don't think he even knew I was there.' The staff nurse had been faced with the same situation herself many times; she knew exactly how to deal with it.

'You'll have to go back with it later then, when he's finished saying his prayers, won't you?' she told the assistant nurse.

'Yes, Staff,' said the assistant, still looking puzzled. It wasn't always easy for a busy nurse to wait patiently for a devout Hindu to finish saying his prayers before she could give him his medicine or injection.

Neither was it easy to know what to do with the sick little Sikh boy's topknot when he was first admitted. That it had some religious meaning we knew, but whether it would jeopardize his soul if one not of his own faith touched it we didn't know, so we left it alone until his mother told us it would be all right, but even then we approached it gingerly.

We had to learn what to do if a Muslim died and, just as important, what not to do if a Hindu died. I remembered a very long time ago, when I wasn't a staff nurse, being on a ward where a man who had died was not of a faith we were familiar with. We had proceeded with the usual last offices only to discover when it was too late that we shouldn't have touched him at all. It took his relatives and their religious advisers several hours to undo the damage we had done. They sluiced him down in the yard outside the ward window with water from a hose attached to the kitchen tap. I was very glad I was only a probationer at the time and didn't have to go to the Matron's office to be told off for not knowing how to go about such things. Knowledge like that was supposed to come naturally to nurses.

Lynch made a terrible mistake one night while she was working on the cubicle wards. When the handsome, bearded giant of a Sikh told her he was hungry because he hadn't eaten his supper that night, she didn't stop to ask him if there was any particular reason why he hadn't eaten his supper. She gave him a long, yearning look of compassion, and then rushed to the kitchen and made him a tremendous corned beef sandwich to appease his hunger. While she was making it she hinted that she would be almost tempted to give him more than a corned beef sandwich to appease any other hungers he might have. We reminded her sharply that as well as being a married woman she was a Catholic and he was a Sikh, and the Pope would never stand for such an alliance. She finished the sandwich and took it down to the Sikh. She told us about it when she got back to the kitchen.

'He was ever so grateful for it until he saw what was between the bread,' she said sadly, tipping the sandwich into the pedal bin. 'Then he nearly threw it at me. He doesn't eat cow, he says. I didn't know corned beef was cow. It doesn't even taste like beef anyway.'

I should have learned a lesson from Lynch's experience but I didn't. When the same Sikh asked me to find him something to read I searched through the bookshelf at home and eventually chose a book I had enjoyed reading. It was well written, amusing and factual. I gave it to him that night and he glanced briefly at the jacket, took in the gaudy gory Spanish scene and handed me back the book. 'And why would a Sikh be interested in the bull fight?' he asked with tremendous dignity. Why indeed? Gentle creature as the cow is to a Westerner and exciting challenge that the bull is to a Spaniard, nowhere are they held in as much reverence as they are in India. I hurried out of the cubicle as Lynch had done, taking my offering with me.

But the frightened young girls we got in were even more of a problem than the men who were particular about their food. The girls had only just arrived in the strange cold country that was England, and had no idea what was happening to them or what was going to happen to them next. Some had been sent from home to marry boys they had never seen, but even that couldn't have been as frightening for them as being surrounded by a bunch of women who insisted on them eating things they had no appetite for and kept doing things to them that were sometimes very painful. When they were too tired even to cry any more they turned their faces to the wall and refused to listen while we were trying to tell them that the things we did for them were for their benefit and not ours. This is something which even patients who speak the same language as their nurses often find hard to understand.

The young Asian girls were not the only ones to weep and stare at blank walls. When a Turkish mother and her two small children were brought in one night, she refused to be separated from the children. She didn't understand one word of what we were saying to her, and we were just as helpless.

'We'll have to put a couple of cot beds in her cubicle for the children,' said the night sister. This was usually only done when two children of one family were admitted with the same complaint; only very rarely were there ever three beds in a cubicle. We pushed and shoved for the next half hour, taking cots out of cubicles where there were no patients and manoeuvring them into the Turkish lady's cubicle. After it was all done we stood and tried to explain to her that the cots were for her children. When at last she understood she shook her head fiercely, put the children one on either side of her in her own bed and sat up all night staring fixedly at the opposite wall while they slept the sleep they so badly needed after their flight from Turkey. For the three days and nights they were in she refused to let anybody but herself touch either of her children. We were very happy that none of them had the thing the airport doctor thought they had. Three in a bed for three nights was headache enough for us, but three in a bed for the duration of a protracted infectious disease would have played havoc with our routine. None of us liked such deviation from the norm.

But the saddest of all our immigrant patients were the very young children. They stood in a corner of their cots screaming for things they had no name for that we could understand. We plonked them on potties when it was a drink they wanted and plied them with drinks when they were crying for their mummies. They were small bundles of misery for whom we had no word of comfort.

'Why their mothers can't teach them a word or two of English before they come into hospital I really don't know,' said the menopausal sister, driven to hot flushes of frustration by one of the uncomprehending children. She knew as well as we did that the reason their mothers didn't teach them a word or two of English was because they didn't know a single word of English themselves. It would take a year or two before the children started teaching their mothers their new language.

There were other, less harrowing, aspects of the language difficulties. We quickly discovered that the first few words of English that many of the immigrant men learned were often the more indelicate ones. This aptitude for acquiring a vocabulary not usually heard in polite society confused even me one night.

I had gone to answer a bell, after waiting long enough to make sure that nobody else was going to answer it. The man who had rung the bell had only been admitted earlier that evening from the airport. He looked very tired and very lost.

'What did you ring for?' I asked him, speaking in the loud and very distinct tones that English people use when they are talking to foreigners. The man in the bed twiddled nervously with his pyjama cord.

'I need peace,' he said.

For a moment I thought he was delirious, but there had been nothing in the day staff's report to suggest any sudden deterioration in his condition. He was in with a simple suspected infection that should have caused nobody any anxiety.

'Try and go to sleep,' I said, giving him a kind little smile to put his mind at rest in case he thought I was saying something nasty.

'I need peace,' he repeated, twiddling the pyjama

cord again but this time in a very agitated way. At that moment the night sister came into the cubicle. I was happy to see her; I was already out of my depth.

'He says he needs peace,' I whispered to her. 'I haven't got a clue what he means.' She grinned at me and went out through the door again. She came back with something that she handed to the man.

'Is this what you want?' she asked him in a perfectly normal voice. He grabbed the bottle off her and stuffed it down his bed. A look of relief came over his face.

'I peace now,' he said gratefully.

After that, whenever one of the immigrants told me he needed peace I knew it was not the peace that passeth all understanding that he craved. Even the word 'sheet' when gasped out by a man whose grasp of the English language was minimal seldom meant that he was gasping for bed linen; it almost always indicated that unless we fetched him a bedpan without delay we would all be in trouble.

The man who had begged for peace was a nice man. We were sorry when he went out. Despite his basic English he made up for whatever he couldn't say by giving us beaming smiles, and eloquent and sometimes embarrassing gestures. The day staff told us that on the morning he was discharged a taxi came to the ward door and more than a dozen of his relatives fell out of it. The reunion on the forecourt was very emotional, and when the last tear had been wiped away and the final beam given to the nursing staff everybody including the ex-patient bundled back into the taxi and off they went to the West Midlands, where the streets were also bright with saris and turbans. It must have cost an awful lot of money to hire a taxi from the West Midland Mecca all the way to our fever hospital and back to the West Midlands again, but no expense was ever spared to make the touching reunions on the fore-court worthy of those who had just landed at London Airport.

Soon we were getting in so many immigrant patients that a bungalow had to be built in the grounds to accommodate mothers and children who were only there until their quarantine period was over. Lynch sighed when she saw the bungalow taking shape. 'That's just the sort of place I need,' she said. 'It would be a lot nicer than living in a Nissen hut.' She never got such a splendid residence, but she did get a council house after she had had enough babies to earn her the necessary points. Having to have babies before she could get a proper house to put them in seemed to Lynch a very Irish way of going about things.

The bungalow in the grounds was a mixed blessing. It left the cubicles empty for more needy cases but put a great deal of extra responsibility on the night staff. We had to keep a sharp ear open for sounds of taxis drawing up outside. The men from the West Midlands or even from the nearby town had waited a long time for their loved ones to join them, having to wait another three weeks until the quarantine period was over could put a tremendous strain on a devoted father or a lusty young husband. We had long and noisy arguments, punctuated with plenty of telling gestures, while we were trying to persuade husbands and fathers to climb back into their taxis and wait a little longer for the reunion. We never lost an argument, but we had to use endless diplomacy and exactly the right gestures to win them. The men had come with the intention of snatching their loved ones and going off with them into the night; having to go empty-handed caused them great sorrow. We understood their sorrow, but we thought of all the smallpox that could be let loose if we allowed them to win the arguments.

We didn't get the chance to argue with the men who came to snatch away the beautiful Indian girl with tuberculosis. When the doctor told her about the tuberculosis and said she would have to go to another hospital until her lungs were healed, she turned her face to the wall and wouldn't even look up when we tried to tempt her with the finest hospital cuisine. She had heard of other immigrants who were discovered to have tuberculosis; she knew that she could be put on to a plane and sent straight back home instead of being allowed to stay and marry the boy her parents had chosen for her with the help of their local marriage broker. And if she had to be in another hospital while her lungs were healed who was to say that the boy who had been in England for almost a year might not have become so Westernized that he would be looking else-where for a bride? The thought was too painful to be endured, so she kept her face turned to the wall.

But the chosen bridegroom had seen pictures of his future bride. He liked what he saw so much that he and his brothers hired a taxi one night and when every nurse was busy in some other cubicle they whisked her away, tubercular lungs and all. It was doubtful whether there would ever be any marriage. If the tuberculosis didn't catch up with the girl the immigration authorities would.

Another of our lusty young men didn't snatch his wife from her bed or bundle her into a taxi. He rushed her up the corridor and bundled her into the bathroom. And right under the very noses of the day staff.

For several visiting times before he did the rushing and bundling, the young man had been observed through the observation porthole in the cubicle door doing things with his bed-bound little wife that the day sister didn't strictly approve of. She had been glueing her scandalized eye to the porthole for several minutes before she finally burst in one evening and ruined things for them. Though she didn't exactly say 'you can't do that there 'ere', she made enough gestures and stormed loudly enough to convey to the young man that he was breaking the law – her law at least. He rose from the bed reluctantly.

'But she is my wife,' he said. 'I do only the things that the law allows.' His plea got him nowhere. The sister issued her ultimatum. Either he kept out of the bed or he kept out of the cubicle, he could choose for himself.

The following evening, the nurse whose duty it was to check the portholes to see that nothing exciting was happening gave a small scream. The cubicle was empty. Another nurse who had heard the small scream came along to see what it was all about.

'They've eloped,' gasped the first nurse, forgetting that the couple who should have been in the cubicle were already married. They flung open the door to make sure that no forbidden act was going on where the view from the porthole couldn't reach. There wasn't a soul in sight. The birds had flown.

'What are we going to tell Sister?' they asked each other, knowing how the sister felt about patients who took their own discharge when her back was turned. Luckily they didn't have to tell the sister. The man in the next cubicle opened his door an inch and told them what had happened.

'The last I saw of them they were belting up the corridor towards the bathroom,' he said gleefully. 'If you hurry you might get there before it's too late.' It was too late. A bath might not be the most convenient place in a hospital ward to satisfy hunger, but when the nurses entered without even knocking the two hungry little people from Bangladesh looked well satisfied.

The man in the next cubicle said he didn't blame the young man for having a bit of how's your father in the bath. He would have done the same himself, he said, but his old woman wasn't such a good looker as the Indian girl, so he could afford to wait until he got home.

When holidays on the Costa Brava started to be as much within the reach of the masses as cars and telephones, a different type of infectious disease began to find its way into our cubicles. It was something which only the fever-trained nurses had first-hand experience of; the rest of us had only read about typhoid fever in textbooks, and listened to lectures on it given to us by our sister tutors. I had had a question on it when I sat my finals and gave quite the wrong answer, so my knowledge of it was limited. Hitherto the closest we had come to anything akin to typhoid was when a restaurant was closed down in the town after mice droppings were found in the flour. But salmonella wasn't nearly as serious as typhoid, though it kept us busy for several weeks.

The patients who came in with the disease were usually young enough or adventurous enough to risk spending anything up to forty pounds on one of the new package tours that promised two weeks of glorious sunshine but said nothing about the many weeks that might be spent in a fever hospital with typhoid when the holiday was over. Some of the patients were parents who had taken their children on holiday with them. This made the horror of coming home with typhoid even more horrendous.

We had just started to accept the horror as an annual hazard, keeping us extra busy while the summer was at its height and the charter planes were full, when Margaret and her baby son were admitted, both with confirmed typhoid, and both very dangerously ill.

For a long time Margaret lay too close to death to know that her son was struggling to live in one of the cubicles further up the corridor, and we went off duty in the morning tired and anxious and came back again in the evening still tired and just as anxious.

'How's Margaret?' we asked before we even got into the office to read the report book and find out for ourselves how Margaret was. When we were told that Margaret had survived another day, we asked just as fearfully how the baby was. When we were told that he also had survived, we had a quick look through the portholes to see if they were telling us the truth, and only then did we go to the office to get the official verdict of their condition.

Because we were all afraid that the day might come when Margaret would have to be told that there was no little boy for her to go home to we kept up a conspiracy of silence to ensure that she never even suspected that he was no more than three cubicles away from her. Her husband conspired with us. He came in every evening on his way from work, put on a gown and mask and sat beside her bed, telling her happy little stories about the child who had just had his first birthday. He told her lies about the one flickering candle on the birthday cake and all the lovely presents he had played with afterwards. And he told the lies so convincingly that Margaret believed him and shed a few tears because she hadn't been at home for her son's first birthday. But he held her hand tightly and told her not to worry; there would be plenty more birthdays when they would all be together for her to help blow out the candles. Then he took off the gown and mask, washed his hands and went down the corridor to put on another gown and mask and sit beside his son's cot.

The moralists among us who are opposed to telling a lie for whatever reason might have found the situation easier to deal with than we did. Feeling in duty bound to tell the truth, the whole truth and nothing but the truth might have been less of a strain than having to skirt round the truth so that nobody would get hurt by knowing it. The shock of discovering what we were trying to hide from Margaret would have caused her a great deal of unhappiness, and may even have undone a lot of the good that the antibiotics were slowly but surely doing.

As the weeks went by, both mother and son began to get better, he more quickly than she. Soon he was strong enough to hang over the sides of his cot demanding the things that had been denied him over the weeks. He demanded a lot of things in a very loud voice. Being a patient so long among a lot of part-time nurses who were mothers themselves had turned him into a very impatient little boy, but we gave him most of the things he asked for, only too glad that at last he was well enough to scream for them. We told ourselves that we were there to nurse him and not to tell him what a naughty baby he was. We left the corrective treatment for his mother to do when they were both at home again, and tried not to think of the sleepless nights she and his father would have while he hung over the sides of his cot shrieking for biscuits.

Once when a cubicle door was carelessly left open, Margaret looked at the nurse who was blanket bathing her.

'I can hear that baby again,' she said, her eyes brimming with tears. 'I've heard him before. It always makes me think of my little boy at home.'

The nurse turned Margaret over to wash her back and the conspiracy of silence went on.

When at last we started asking each other and the good Jewish doctor whether the time had come for her to be told, something always seemed to crop up to put off the telling for a while longer: Margaret's temperature shot up again for some reason, Margaret had a fit of depression or some other little something happened to her to make it wiser to put off telling her the truth for yet another few days. It was Mother's Day before it was finally agreed she was strong enough to hear that her little boy was only three cubicles away from her. But none of us had to tell her. He told her himself. Again a cubicle door was carelessly – or perhaps deliberately – left open. It was the first time any of us had heard him say 'Mamma'. He said it very clearly. Margaret's bell rang and the conspiracy was over.

'I think maybe I have known all the time,' she said to the nurse who went to answer the bell. 'I just didn't want to let myself believe it.' She laughed through the tears. 'But I shall never trust my husband again. I didn't know he was such a good liar.'

After that, other patients came in with typhoid. There was Diane who was flown back home when she tripped down the holiday hotel steps and broke her arm. Even being brought into us with typhoid didn't stop her from grumbling about breaking her arm when her holiday was only half over.

There was also the Asian family, who came in one by

one and went out one by one, luckily not too much the worse for the mild attack of typhoid they all had, which had been given to them by a Methuselah of an old man who was somebody's great-grandfather, but we never discovered exactly whose great-grandfather he was. He had flown to England with the family, and from the little we were able to gather, had been giving people typhoid fever for a long time.

We nursed so many people over the years with typhoid that whenever we read in the paper that a case of typhoid had been admitted to some hospital or another we thought of our own and were glad nothing was ever published about them in the local papers. There had been enough panic in the town over a single suspected case of smallpox; several confirmed cases of typhoid would have started a stampede.

But the typhoid never became an epidemic. The epidemic that was to fill our cubicles and the new long ward as well was something quite different, and something we knew little about unless we were fever trained, which I was not.

Chapter Seventeen

UNTIL THE TIME that Mr Franklin D. Roosevelt of the United States of America was stricken with infantile paralysis, it was generally supposed that the disease was one which only affected children, hence the name it was known by for many years. Later, when Mr Roosevelt became President of the United States, there seemed something inspiring, if not downright romantic, about a fine handsome man like him being confined to a wheelchair. It gave hope to others who were similarly handicapped. Later still, when the war was on and we saw pictures of the President with Messrs Stalin and Churchill at some very important meeting in Yalta, not only were we stirred by the significance of the meeting but we marvelled at the courage of the man who had learned to live with his afflictions in such distinguished style.

But very much later still when infantile paralysis was given its true name and became popularly known as polio, there was nothing romantic about the epidemic that spread around the country, crippling young men and women, and even the middle-aged as well as children. Those who emerged from it in wheelchairs needed all the inspiring they could get – whether it was from the history of men like President Roosevelt or from more ordinary mortals who had triumphed over their handicap.

When the first few suspected cases of polio started to trickle into our cubicles, all the fears the part-timers had ever had about taking infection home to their families started up again but with greater force. Those who had walked willingly across the grounds from the chronic wards to help out during a temporary emergency thought twice about it when they were asked to come over to relieve until the epidemic died down. Some said they would rather stay with the grannies than watch children die of polio. Others said they were afraid for their own children at home. Nobody was made to come across unless they were employed from the beginning for the fever side. I and others who had weathered the storm of typhoid and a variety of acutely infectious diseases, reasoned that if the rules we kept then were enough to ensure that we didn't pedal any of them home with us, then we could surely nurse polio without endangering our families.

Lynch, who had just come back to work after having special leave to have her second baby, volunteered to work on the cubicles. Her mother had kindly volunteered to mind both the children when Lynch was in bed or on duty.

'You don't *have* to come across to the fever side,' I said to her when she first reported on duty. 'You're an auxiliary and could say you didn't want to because of the children at home.'

Lynch looked at me in some surprise. 'But what if it was my children in here with it? I would hope there were enough nurses on to look after them properly.' She knew as we all knew that the time would come when we would need all the staff we could get on the fever side.

Brown went to the Matron and told her that since she had done some fever nursing in the past she would like to go on the cubicles. I was glad when she reported on duty. I felt that however black things became, she would lighten them for me as she had done before. None of us could have even imagined how black everything would soon become. Suddenly we were witnessing sorrow which even we, accustomed as we were to witnessing sorrow, found ourselves shrinking from. For many of us it was the saddest time of all our nursing career.

Those of us who had never nursed polio before, or ever seen an iron lung in action, looked with horror at the ugly monsters that had been fetched from somewhere in case of emergency. We listened intently while the doctor and the fever-trained sisters told us exactly how to put a patient into one of the lungs, and how to nurse the patients once they were in the lungs; as we listened, we were hoping that the things we were listening to would never have to be done – or if they did and we were called upon to do them there would be somebody on duty with us who knew more about them than we did. But before the epidemic was over we had nursed enough patients in the lungs to be almost as expert at it as the sisters.

We also learned how to manage the hand pump if the electricians suddenly went on strike, or there was a power cut to stop the bellows working. That was something else we hoped would never happen while we were on duty.

Not everybody who was admitted with suspected polio was a confirmed case. The family doctors started playing it safe and begging for beds for anybody who went to their surgeries with a stiff neck, a feverish cold or any slight ache or pain that had come on suddenly for no apparent reason. The stiff neck might only have been the result of the patient sitting in a draught at home, at school or wherever they worked; the feverish cold was often nothing more than a feverish cold; and the aches and pains were frequently caused by an orgy of gardening, housework or something a great deal more pleasant. But they were all sent in to us to be officially diagnosed and have any doubts removed. We were as happy as the patients were when we could tell them that the cold was a cold, the stiff neck only a stiff neck and the nagging little aches and pains the result of orgies. We laughingly told them that whatever orgy they indulged in should be rather less strenuous the next time they indulged in it.

But if the feverish cold was polio after all, we kept them in; and, if nothing happened after three weeks and the cold was better, they went home, glad that they could move their arms and legs freely with no sign even of muscular weakness. If there was muscular weakness, or some paralysis, we splinted and bandaged the paralysed parts and watched anxiously for signs of the paralysis creeping on and into chest muscles, making it necessary for another lung to be brought to the ward. And if the lung was needed, we listened all night to the bellows pumping breath into lungs that could no longer draw their own breath.

If the doctor in charge of the cubicles had been a rock for us to lean on before the polio epidemic broke out, now he was the strength that kept us going when we felt we couldn't go on a minute longer. He was on call night and day, snatching as much sleep as he could between calls. At whatever hour we needed him he heaved himself out of bed and came to the cubicles, or to the new long ward that had to be opened, wearing an assortment of clothing that included such diverse things as a pair of flying boots, jazzy pyjamas, a long black coat and a round black hat. The hat was only worn at certain times, and we could never be certain if it had a religious significance or whether it was simply put on to keep his bald patch warm.

He only once came to the cubicles in the night attired in a fashion becoming to a doctor and a gentleman. He arrived in a state of unsuppressed excitement. His dress was faultless, his linen spotless. We hardly recognized him.

When we expressed surprise at seeing him there, since nobody had sent for him, he gave a smirk of false modesty and spread out his hands in a very Jewish way.

'I've been summoned by the Duchess,' he said, naming a Royal and very gracious lady who lived in a modest residence not far from the hospital. 'It seems that the Prince has a slight sore throat and his personal physician is away for the night.' He made it sound like a scene from a musical comedy, but we were deeply impressed by the honour that had been conferred upon him.

After he had graciously accepted our congratulations, he went down the corridor to the medical room and gathered together enough antibiotics, dressings and sore-throat cures to treat the entire Royal Family. Then he straightened his tie, rubbed his bald patch and went to obey the Royal Command.

We heard no more about the very important sore throat he had gone out in the night to cure but, as there were no bulletins posted outside Buckingham Palace, we could only assume his mission had been successful. For a day or two after that, he went round looking as if he was expecting to receive a knighthood, and then the memory of his brief hour of glory faded and he started coming to the ward in his flying boots again.

As well as being good with Royal sore throats, he had a wonderful way with slipped discs. However far they had managed to slip, he could put them back into place with one swift and very painful manipulation. I only saw him do it once, but it left a permanent scar on my memory.

When the night sister came on duty one evening looking tired and ill and complaining of pains somewhere round the back of her chest, we made sympathetic noises and told her that she should have stayed at home and gone to bed instead of coming to work. We were very glad she hadn't stayed at home and gone to bed; we were far too busy to be minus a night sister, especially one who worked as hard as she did.

We went over her symptoms one by one, then told her that in our opinion she was suffering from pleurisy. She thanked us for our optimistic diagnosis and continued to suffer bravely for the next three hours. When the doctor came on the ward at midnight to see a new patient, we showed him the night sister as well. He went over her symptoms one by one, and then told her that in his opinion she was suffering from a slipped disc. He refused the stethoscope I was offering him to go over the chest the sister had already bared for his inspection, and invited her to sit down on a kitchen chair. Then he pinioned her arms behind her back and pulled. What he pulled we didn't know – the movement was too swift to follow – but the sister gave a terrible yell, leapt out of the chair and was cured.

Afterwards, whenever I thought of the sister's yell, I prayed it would never be my misfortune to slip a disc while our doctor was around. Dying with pleurisy would surely have been less agonizing. But sometimes, when I read about the number of working hours lost by men who were chronic backache sufferers, I got the feeling that if they had heard the yell, and were promised the same remedial treatment for their backache, they might have preferred to return quietly to work and endure their sufferings with more fortitude.

However tired we nurses were during the polio epidemic, we knew that the doctor was just as tired. No sooner was he back in bed after easing our mind about one desperately ill patient than he was hurling himself out of it again to see another who had just been admitted. Nevertheless, though I sympathized with his tiredness and was grateful to him for his never-failing kindness and courtesy, even I was astonished one night when I pushed a laid-up trolley into a cubicle and found him in bed with the beautiful blonde who had just come in to have her stiff neck diagnosed.

Lynch, who was following me with a pile of clean towels and pillow cases, stopped dead at the door. 'Holy Mother of God!' she exclaimed wildly, trying to cross herself and dropping the towels in the attempt. Like me she had an instant vision of the double-spread scandal the Sunday papers would make of it when the beautiful young woman sued the doctor for professional misconduct – though she was certainly showing no sign of resenting his intrusion into her bed. She even looked as if she might be enjoying it. He was a very personable man.

He looked at us and beamed – he also seemed to be enjoying the position he was in. He was wearing his black hat that night and hadn't got round to removing it.

'Don't worry, it's all perfectly respectable,' he said, making it all seem perfectly respectable. 'I was just asking her if she could kiss her knees and she said she could but she doubted very much whether I would be able to kiss mine. I was just showing her that I could.' He kissed his knees again for our benefit, and then climbed from the bed, getting the heel of his flying boot caught up in the counterpane.

We accepted his account of the incident and watched him while he did a lumbar puncture that was a more reliable test for polio than the knee-kissing one, though that had its uses as an early indication of how stiff the neck was.

Later, when Lynch, the night sister and I were snatching a quick midnight meal in the kitchen Lynch referred to the doctor's unorthodox conduct.

'I wonder why he never gets into bed with the men when they come in with a stiff neck,' she said thoughtfully.

'Perhaps it's because they never challenge him to kiss his knees,' said the sister. 'And anyway, it wouldn't be nearly as much fun climbing into bed with the men, do you think?' She was also Irish and as devout a Catholic as Lynch. Once, when somebody brought in a bag of hot-cross buns for our Good Friday supper, the cross on her bun had slid off the sugar-glazed top and landed on the floor.

'Jesus, Mary and Joseph, it's detachable crosses now,' she said, staring down at the mass-produced plastic-looking thing that lay at her feet. We were still more used to the crosses on our hot-cross buns being inden-tations in the dough that the bun was made from. Detachable crosses were only just finding their way into the hot-cross bun industry.

Lynch pondered for a moment on what the night sister had said about how dull it would be for the doctor to climb into bed with the men. 'No, I suppose you're right, it wouldn't be much fun for him,' she said, nibbling her starch-reduced crispbread. We were all on a very strict diet that night. The strict one we'd been on the night before hadn't worked at all.

The beautiful young woman didn't have polio, neither did she sue the doctor for professional misconduct. She had been too pleased that her stiff neck was only a stiff neck to mind one of his flying boots getting caught up in her counterpane.

But she was one of the lucky ones. Others were not so lucky. Some were very unlucky indeed. New young mothers were brought in, wondering how long it would be before they saw their new little baby again, or any of the other children they had left behind them at home. They also wondered whether any of the children, or even the new little baby, would develop the symptoms that had brought them into the fever hospital. Worrying about that did nothing to help their recovery. Mothers-to-be came in fearing what might happen to the baby they had been so eagerly awaiting. Those who were already severely paralysed knew that if the baby was delivered successfully it would be through the surgeon's skill in the theatre rather than their own labours in the delivery room. Middle-aged mums were admitted worrying about the housework they had left unfinished at home, and dads were rushed in dreading that the legs that felt numb and useless would go on feeling numb and useless for a long time, if not for ever.

Parents stood looking down at their splinted and padded children and could scarcely believe that it was only yesterday that they had complained of a sore throat, or of feeling hot when they should have been feeling cold, or simply hadn't wanted to go to school and had to be reminded sternly that it was nearly nine o'clock and they'd better get a move on before they got a black mark for being late – and no, they couldn't take a note to the teacher asking to be excused games. Nobody knew enough about polio then to know that if *only* people had stopped doing the things they were doing *the moment* the virus infection struck they might just have been spared being paralysed by it. The middle-aged mum who died in the lung might not even have died if only she had stopped polishing the floors when she felt too ill to lift a duster. It was important for her to get the polishing done, especially if she was going to be ill; it would never do to let the doctor come and find the house less than spotless. Even when the funny sensation she had first felt in her arms started to creep into her chest she went on polishing. When her husband came home in the evening he found her lying on the floor still in her pinny and with the duster beside her. She apologized for there being no dinner on the table and begged him to tidy the bedroom before the doctor came. She was only in a lung for a few hours, then the bellows were the only things in the cubicle that were making any sound.

The athletic young man who came into her cubicle after she died would never move either of his legs again. He had insisted on batting for his side even though he had a sore throat and a slightly stiff neck. He didn't make a century because, as the game progressed, he found it harder to run from one set of stumps to the other.

'What will he do?' his mother asked us, when she stumbled out of the cubicle while we were splinting and padding his legs and putting sandbags at his feet in order to prevent foot drop. The young man didn't do anything. He just lay there letting us do it all for him. He cried a lot, especially after his mates from the cricket club came to see him. Soon they stopped coming to see him; it was hard to make conversation with a man who resented them having two good legs to walk on when he had lost the use of his.

But not everybody was as defeated as he was. Some of our patients cried a lot at first, then stopped crying and got down to the business of building a new life for themselves.

When Maureen was admitted to the second cubicle from the medical room, she told us that the doctor who assured her that the feverish cold she had was a touch of flu was as surprised as she was when her legs buckled beneath her and she had more than a touch of polio. She was young and pretty and pregnant. It was a long time before her legs were able to support her properly again, but when her baby was born it screamed as hard and as healthily as if its mother hadn't got polio at all. Years later when we saw Maureen in the town with her four fine children, it was hard to believe that we had once doubted whether she would ever be able to walk again. We barely noticed that she went over a little on one side and sometimes needed a stick to help her along. Having a pram to push must have given her strength as well as courage. She needed all she could get of both when she went out of the second cubicle from the medical room.

David was another young man who cried a lot at first. He was fine and handsome, six feet tall and the breadwinner in his family. His mother was a widow with three sons younger than David, and he was only twenty. Having her eldest son paralysed from the waist down with a bit of weakness in his arms as well wasn't going to make life any easier for her.

Every morning on the dot of six she telephoned from a kiosk, on her way to the office-cleaning job she did, to ask how David was. We would tell her that his condition remained unchanged and that he was comfortable, and she would go to work knowing at least that he was no worse than he was the last time she phoned or came to see him. Being told that a patient is comfortable doesn't necessarily mean that the patient thinks he is comfortable; it more often than not simply indicates that the patient isn't rolling on the bed in agony.

On the morning that David's mother didn't ring on the dot of six, we told him she had and wondered why she hadn't. We were just starting to visualize her being mown down by an early morning bus, or foully murdered by a maniac, when the phone rang and it was her.

'Sorry I didn't ring sooner,' she shrieked almost loudly enough for us to hear her without the intermediary of the telephone. 'There was this drunk propped up in the phone box, see, so I shut the door quick and ran down the road like hell. It gave me quite a turn I might tell you, finding a drunk propped up in the phone box. How's David this morning?' We told her that David remained comfortable and said that it would have given us quite a turn as well if we had found a drunk propped up in the phone box at six o'clock in the morning. I had once found a man-sized plaster cast propped up in a moonlit lavatory, and it had given me such a turn that I had run away, quite forgetting that nurses were only allowed to run in case of fire or haemorrhage. No exception was made in those days for coming suddenly upon a ghost in the lavatory. I got into a great deal of trouble for so flagrantly breaking the rules.

David went out in a wheelchair, leaving us all a little sad but, knowing how quickly he had stopped crying over the milk that was spilt and would never be mopped up again, we had every faith in him as a top challenger in the wheelchair race. And though his mother might have run like hell from the drunk in the phone box, she would make it her business to see that David didn't run away from anything, which was very important for a man who was paralysed from the waist down.

We had grown very tired of comforting heart-broken mothers, switching off lungs when the patients in them would no longer benefit from the action of the bellows, and seeing young men like David go home in wheel-chairs, when Reg came in to bring us all to the brink of despair. Even nurses can stand only so much sadness. If it goes on too long they start to fray at the edges and wallow in the sadness in spite of everything their sister tutors ever taught them about not bleeding too much for their patients. It was impossible for any of us to stay cool and detached about Reg.

Part Six

Chapter Eighteen

REG WAS IN a lung for a long time. We took it in turns to watch over him while he gasped in rhythm to the gasping bellows. He spent the greater part of every night telling us naughty stories which took him so long to tell that we usually lost the point before the punch line was even in sight. But afterwards, each of his stories was included in our repertoire of naughty stories – not so much because they were funny, or even very naughty, but because of his unique way of telling them: 'Have (gasp) you (gasp) heard (gasp) this one (gasp), nurse?' Often we had but we said we hadn't. The stories kept Reg's mind off his numb legs, useless arms and no-good chest muscles.

Sometimes, when he wasn't keeping us convulsed with his stories, he told us little anecdotes about his three children, and we told him little anecdotes about ours, and when at last he closed his eyes and we knew he was asleep we stayed awake in spite of our tiredness and watched for anything that would warn us to reach for the emergency bell. We also spent time going over in our minds what to do if the electricians came out on a lightning strike. So far they never had, but there was always a first time for everything.

Reg's wife visited him as often as she could get somebody to look after the children. She breezed into his cubicle, put on her gown and mask and sat beside the lung while she told her husband how well they were managing at home without him. Then, when it was time for her to leave, she would stand for a moment leaning against the wall outside the cubicle, and we could see by her face that they weren't managing at all well without him.

When he was at last able to breathe for a moment or two without the lung he was taken out of it for a little longer each day.

On his birthday he sat in a chair for half an hour, and that night he died.

I was on duty when it happened. We waited for a long time before we switched off the lung. The doctor said it was no use keeping it running any longer, but there seemed something murderous in stopping the breathing, even if it was only mechanical breathing caused by the bellows of the lung.

When everything was done that had to be done, I went and stood at the office window and wondered why I was there at all. I wanted to go home and leave the dying for others to cope with. I was tired of finding comforting things to say to people who in the end would have to find their own comfort no matter what I said. I just wanted to get on my bicycle and pedal away down the road. Then suddenly a bird started to sing outside the window, soon others joined in and the sweetness of the dawn chorus took my mind off the harshness of other things. I listened and felt better. I was grateful to the birds for waking up just when I needed them.

Nothing was ever quite so bad after that night. Patients still came in with polio but none of them had to go into a lung, and those who were paralysed would be able to walk again and even work again, after weeks of massage and exercise and rehabilitation at the place that was specially equipped for such things.

Ragnor and the very rich lady were two of our last polio patients. Ragnor was a Norwegian. He was blond and gorgeous. He had come to London to marry the girl he met when he came to London the year before. Instead of his best man taking him to church, he took him to a doctor who said he had polio and sent him in to us. We breathed a sigh of relief as the days went by and nothing too terrible happened to him. When he went out looking little the worse for his three weeks' stay, he invited us all to the postponed wedding – but none of us went; we were all too tired.

The very rich lady couldn't move at all when she was first admitted, but she could still talk. When she realized that she had been transferred from an expensive private clinic to a free National Health hospital she was extremely upset. She would have walked out at once except that both her legs were useless. Instead she listened while the doctor used his charm on her and told her that the expensive private clinic she had been transferred from didn't have an iron lung, should she be unfortunate enough to need one; neither did it have the facilities for nursing acutely infectious diseases, despite the astronomical fees it charged merely for allowing a patient to enter the front door. He also told her that National Health doctors, and National Health nurses, were really not so bad if only she would give us a chance to prove it. She succumbed to his charms and, instead of finding fault with everything we did as she had looked like doing when she first came in, she let us get on with anything we had to do and even thanked us for doing it. She went home with very different views on the National Health Service than she had when she was admitted. She also had two strong legs, which was more than she came in with.

When the polio epidemic was finally over and the cubicles were again filled with acutely infectious liver complaints, glandular fever and all the other complaints that had filled them before the polio victims took possession, the doctor who had been our rock invited us into the committee room one evening. He had already had the day staff in the committee room earlier. He said such nice things about us and the team-work of the past months that we had to pretend it was the weak gin and orange we were drinking that was making us so sentimental. We had caviar and other things with the gin and orange.

'What's this?' asked Lynch, spooning some of the caviar on to a biscuit.

'It's caviar,' we told her, trying to make it sound as if we ate it every day. She took a tiny taste and spat it out.

'I don't like it,' she said, washing her mouth round with some more gin and orange. 'It's salty and it tastes nasty and it looks like tapioca pudding, only black.'

None of us liked it much but we ate it nevertheless. It made a change from the usual things we ate, and it seemed rude to go straight on to the sausage rolls and vol-au-vents, especially after the doctor had gone to such trouble to provide it for us.

But though the polio was no longer in our cubicles except for an occasional suspect who turned out not to have it, or somebody who did have it but only mildly, we were reminded of the bad times often in the years after.

When a new little apprentice started in the salon where I went when my unmanageable hair had grown more than usually unmanageable, I noticed she had a slight limp. After she had shampooed me a few times, I asked her in a roundabout way how she got the limp.

'I had polio when I was two,' she said. 'I was in the fever hospital for weeks.' I felt a little surge of pride that I might have been one of the nurses who had helped with the padding and splinting so that the limp was no worse. I listened to her while she shampooed me and was glad that the boys noticed her face before they allowed the limp to bother them. According to her she was much in demand at the local dance hall.

The very first time I saw Maureen standing on her own two feet, though not very steadily, I tried to find words to tell her how I felt about her courage.

'You're a clever girl, aren't you?' I said, and she understood perfectly what I meant.

David's mother sent a Christmas card every year, and part-timers who lived near to him said he was still as cheeky as he had always been. Having to live his life in a wheelchair hadn't cramped his style too much.

The very rich lady kept in touch, and invited our rock, our strength, our beautiful Jewish doctor to dinner quite often. We always knew when he had been invited: he came on the ward attired as a doctor and a gentleman, his dress faultless, his linen spotless. It was almost as if he had been summoned again by the Duchess.

The others who didn't keep in touch, either because they had died or because they were too busy doing their remedial exercises, we still thought about and talked about while we were eating our midnight meals in the kitchen. An epidemic of polio isn't quickly forgotten, even by nurses.

The cosy little chats we had in the kitchen weren't nearly as cosy as they had once been. Our children were growing up, and far too fast for most of us. The girls were asking Father Christmas for many-tiered stiffened can-can petticoats to wear themselves instead of diminutive garments to dress their dollies in. They pleaded to be allowed to wear outrageous iridescent socks with Elvis embroidered up the sides. When we insisted on them wearing the snowy white socks which we said looked so much nicer than the iridescent ones they sulked and said that all the other girls at school wore them when they weren't at school, so why shouldn't they? We didn't really know why they shouldn't except that we didn't think they were quite nice. They reminded us that 'niceness' was rapidly going out of fashion; they didn't want to be 'nice', they wanted to be 'mod' like every other girl. There were many battles fought over their right to be like every other girl. They got their can-can petticoats, but they didn't get iridescent socks with Elvis written on them. There had to be a line drawn somewhere!

The part-timers who were mothers of boys had problems as well. Their sons were now 'teenagers' and felt deprived if they weren't allowed to spend the money they saved from paper-round wages on such things as drain-pipe trousers, draped jackets with velvet collars and heavy crepe-soled shoes. The shoes were acceptable – they didn't wear out as quickly as expensive leather ones – but the rest of the uniform that the boys demanded was as revolutionary as iridescent socks, winkle-picker shoes and beehive hairdos.

Some of the boys went to the barber's shop on Saturday morning looking neat and tidy and a credit to their mother's nagging and came out with their hair done in a greasy quiff in the front and something they called a DA at the back.

'I asked him what a DA was,' sobbed a heartbroken mother one night while she and I were admitting Georgie and Sally. Georgie had a glass eye. He was only four. Whenever he wanted to annoy his sister Sally, who was three, he took out the eye and threw it at her. We spent a lot of time in the cubicle where we had doubled them up because they were brother and sister and were both in with the same complaint. Most of the time was spent on our hands and knees looking for Georgie's eye, while he watched us with his one good eye and the hole where the other should have been. He probably didn't realize that he was throwing the glass eye at Sally in anger because she had thrown something at him one day which struck him in the eye and stayed there. That would be kept from him until later, when it would perhaps be a psychiatrist's job to tell him.

'What did he say a DA was?' I asked the heartbroken mother while I popped Georgie's eye back into place.

'He said it stood for the rear end of a duck,' she said, pushing Sally down in her cot and putting up the sides with a bang. 'What things are coming to these days I really don't know.' And neither did I. We read with horror of the goings-on in one of the local cinemas after a so-called 'Rock' film had been shown. The flea-bitten seats had been slashed with knives, and the poor manager was powerless to stop the rampage. The rock-and-rolling Bill Haley and the gyrating Elvis brought out the primitive in his patrons. It wasn't safe to go to the pictures any more, said the staid old picture-goers.

When Shirl came to be a domestic on one of the cubicle wards, the day sister in charge of it temporarily went out of her mind. She had been used to domestics like Lottie. Shirl wasn't a bit like Lottie. She was a teenager, a mod and one of the rock-and-rollers who, if she didn't slash seats in the cinema, loved the boys who did. She came on duty in the morning bleary-eyed with being out so late the night before and still in her beehive hairdo. The beehive was brassy yellow with strawberry-coloured streaks. It towered a good ten inches above her head.

'How do you manage to get it up like that?' we asked her, looking at the mat that hadn't had a comb through it for several days.

'It's back combing,' she said proudly. 'If you back comb it enough it doesn't have to be touched until it's washed. A proper beehive can last for a week.' Hers sometimes looked as if it had lasted for much longer than a week.

When Shirl had been more than usually carried away the night before at a notorious dance hall in the town, she would stand in the kitchen doing energetic movements to the rhythm of the rock music that still rang in her head.

'Whatever are you doing?' we asked her one morning when we went into the kitchen just after she came on duty and just before we were going off. Shirl was standing beside the sink, her fists clenched and alternately crossing her arms and banging her clenched fists down on her knees. She was muttering some curious sort of incantation. There was a glazed look in her eyes.

'One potato, two potatoes, three potatoes, four,' she muttered, increasing the tempo of the knee-banging.

We waited for her to come out of the trance, then we asked her what she thought she was doing when she should have been washing up the breakfast things.

'It's hand jiving,' she said. 'You ought to try it some-time, it really sends you.'

We tried it but it didn't send us. All it did for us was to get us thoroughly confused about which fist we should be knocking on which knee on the down beat.

'You're too old,' said Shirl. 'You're past it.'

And we really began to feel that we were.

Lynch left to have her third baby and we gave her a dozen muslin nappies as a leaving present; the council also gave her enough points to entitle her to a council house which was a lot more exciting for her than our muslin nappies.

Then Brown left. Her middle-aged airman bought a pub and told us we would be very welcome to drop in for a pint if we were ever anywhere near Somerset. We never were. Like the patients, the nurses came and went and became only memories, unless they were part-time married women and we bumped into them while we were doing our shopping.

And then it was my turn to leave – and the thought of no longer being part of a hospital as I had been for thirty years made the leaving sad for me, though I had no choice but to leave.

Chapter Nineteen

WHEN THE LETTER arrived telling me that my mother was drawing her money out of the Co-op bank and had started lighting the fire with five-pound notes, my heart sank. That she was wrapping the notes in paper doilies before she lit the fire with them didn't make anything any better. I knew the time had come when she would have to come and live with us. For one or two very bad moments, I resented the burden that was about to fall on my shoulders and thought about the effect it would have on my family. Then I accepted the inevitable, rearranged the furniture and put up a single bed in the sitting room. I was already resigned to it when I got to the depths of Lincolnshire.

The greeting she gave me when she opened the door wasn't unlike the greeting I got when I went home because my father was dying, but this time there was one small difference. She hadn't the least idea who I was.

'Good afternoon,' she said politely after she had stopped the dog from knocking me over. Part of the reason for the dog being there at all was to protect her from strangers; I was a stranger and he greeted me ecstatically, as I was sure he would have greeted me if I had been a burglar instead of the daughter of the house.

'Are you from the church?' my mother asked, straightening her pinny and showing me into the living room. I was just starting to smile at her little joke when I realized she wasn't joking. I told her that I was her daughter and I'd come to take her home with me, but I had to tell her twice before she even listened. She was busy feeding the dog with a plateful of food that had obviously been intended for her own dinner. When at last she heard me she lifted her head proudly and a little angrily.

'I don't need to come and live with you,' she, said holding a dish of rice pudding under the dog's nose. 'I've got a daughter I can go and live with. She should be here any minute now. I had a letter from her this morning telling me she was coming. She would have come before but she is the Matron of one of the biggest hospitals in London, and it's difficult for her to get away.' She searched among the papers on the mantelshelf and found the letter I had written telling her that I was coming to fetch her to live with us. 'There you are, you see,' she said. 'I told you my daughter was coming to fetch me.'

I saw it would be a waste of time trying to get it across to her that I was the only daughter she had. I also decided it would be just as much of a waste of time telling her that

I was a part-time staff nurse at a very small hospital on the outskirts of London and not the Matron of one of the biggest in London. My mother had always had delusions of grandeur about me when she was impressing her friends and the vicar about my amazing progress as a nurse. I had never spoilt her fun by destroying the delusions, and it was too late to start doing it now.

I spent a few days settling her affairs, seeing if there was anything left in the Co-op savings bank, taking her round to say a puzzled farewell to her friends and finding a good home for the dog. I had a dog of my own and instinct told me that my little corgi wouldn't take kindly to having to move over in his basket to make room for a very large Labrador. My mother didn't seem to notice when a farmer came and took the Labrador away to live happily on a farm with lots of other dogs. I remembered that she hadn't seemed to notice that my father's chair was empty when he was dying in hospital. She was obviously blessed with the merciful blind spot that Brown had talked about.

The journey from the depths of Lincolnshire to the outskirts of London took almost five hours, and at the end of it my mother sank into a chair in my kitchen and took off her hat and gloves.

'My goodness, that's been a long walk,' she said, beaming round at us. 'I feel fair worn out with it all. I could do with a nice cup of tea.'

After she had drunk the tea, she put her hat and gloves on again. 'Well, we'd better be getting back now. It's a tidy walk up the lane and it'll be dark soon.' She walked determinedly out of the door I had only just brought her in through, and stood for a moment looking in bewilderment at the stream of traffic pushing and shoving for priority on the road. 'It must be market day,' she said, and then walked to the end of the road with me following her, wondering what was going to happen next. She stopped on the corner and I stopped as well. After looking again in bewilderment at the traffic she turned to me. 'I think it's time we went home, don't you?' she said. And we went home.

I sat her in front of the television set while I got a meal ready. From that day to the day she died she never questioned where she was. She was occasionally amazed at the sudden mushrooming of the houses that had never been in the lane before, but she seemed to accept them as part of an environmental scheme thought up perhaps by the parochial church council as a means of bringing a bit of life to the lane.

She did, however, question many times who I was. But at the end of all her questioning and my attempts at putting the record straight, she was never any wiser. I sometimes wondered if she would have known me better if I had been her own true daughter instead of a fostered child. But whether she would or not, whatever

I did for her I did as if she had been my own true mother.

Though I kept on working for a month or two after she came to live with us, the time inevitably came when I was snatching fewer and fewer winks of sleep during the days when I was on duty at night. Then the time came when I went to work worrying about her and wondering whether I shouldn't be at home caring for her instead of at work caring for other people. The feeling grew stronger until one morning I stood on the mat in the Matron's office, still a little nervous, though not nearly as nervous as I was when I first stood on a Matron's mat, and told her I would have to leave.

At the end of the month I took off my uniform for the last time. It was the end of thirty years of hard work, plenty of sadness, but a lot of happiness thrown in. I felt a little lost as I pedalled away from the hospital. Shutting a door in one's life is never easy, even if there are still plenty of doors left to open. And I knew that I would find other doors.

About the Author

Brought up in Lincolnshire, Evelyn Prentis (real name Evelyn Taws) left home at eighteen to become a nurse. She later moved to London during the war, where she married and raised her family. Like so many other nurses, she went back to hospital and used any spare time she might have had bringing up her children and running her home. Born in 1915, she sadly died in 2001 at the age of eighty-five.

Evelyn published five books about her life as a nurse, and Ebury Press is reissuing them all. *A Nurse in Time*, *A Nurse in Action* and *A Nurse and Mother* are the first three, and the next two books will follow shortly.

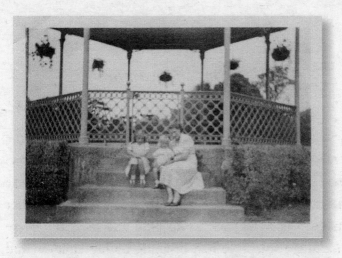

Precious time off-duty for Evelyn, Barbara and Judith.

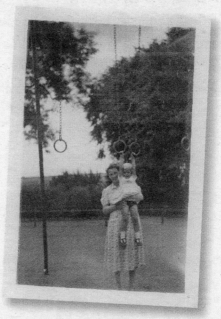

Evelyn and Barbara grappling with Olympic rings, summer 1952.